Fast Facts for Healthcare
Professionals

Epilepsy in Children and Young People

Nicola Heenan RN(Child) BHSc(Hons) PGDip(Epilepsy Care) NIP
Paediatric Lead, Epilepsy Nurses Association (ESNA)
Senior Children's Neurology Nurse Specialist
Hull University Teaching Hospitals NHS Trust
Hull Royal Infirmary
Hull, UK

Kathryn Coleman RN(Child) BA(Hons) PGDip(Epilepsy Care)
Executive Committee Member, Epilepsy Nurses Association (ESNA)
Roald Dahl Paediatric Epilepsy Nurse Specialist
London North West Healthcare NHS Trust
Northwick Park Hospital
London, UK

Phil Tittensor RNLD DipN NIP MSc
Chairperson, Epilepsy Nurses Association (ESNA)
Consultant Nurse for the Epilepsies
The Royal Wolverhampton NHS Trust
Honorary Lecturer, University of Wolverhampton
Wolverhampton, UK

Sheila Shepley RGN BSc PhD
Advanced Nurse Practitioner Clinician
Walton Centre NHS Foundation Trust
Betsi Cadwaladr University Health Board (BCUHB)
Liverpool, UK

Declaration of Independence
This book is as balanced and practical as we can make it.
Ideas for improvement are always welcome: fastfacts@karger.com

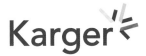

HEALTHCARE

Fast Facts: Epilepsy in Children and Young People
First published 2024

S. Karger Publishers Ltd, Merchant House, 5 East St. Helen Street,
Abingdon, Oxford OX14 5EG, UK

Book orders can be placed by telephone or email, or via the website.
Please telephone +41 61 306 1440 or email orders@karger.com
To order via the website, please go to karger.com

Fast Facts is a trademark of S. Karger Publishers Ltd.

A CIP record for this title is available from the British Library.

ISBN: 978-3-318-07250-1

Heenan N (Nicola)
Fast Facts: Epilepsy in Children and Young People/
Nicola Heenan, Kathryn Coleman, Phil Tittensor, and Sheila Shepley

Illustrations by Graeme Chambers, Belfast, UK.
Typesetting by Amnet, Chennai, India.
Printed in the UK with Xpedient Print.

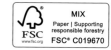

MIX
Paper | Supporting
responsible forestry
FSC® C019670
www.fsc.org

List of abbreviations

ACT: acceptance commitment therapy

ADHD: attention deficit hyperactivity disorder

ALT: alanine transaminase

AMPA: α-amino-3-hydroxy-5-methyl-4-isoxazole propionic acid

ASD: autism spectrum disorder

ASM: antiseizure medication

AV: atrioventricular

bd: twice daily

CAE: childhood absence epilepsy

CBT: cognitive behavioral therapy

CMV: cytomegalovirus

CNS: central nervous system

CT: computed tomography

CYPWE: children and young people with epilepsy

DEE: developmental and/or epileptic encephalopathy

DRN: dorsal raphe nuclei

DS: Dravet syndrome

ECG: electrocardiogram

EEG: electroencephalography/electroencephalogram

GABA: γ-aminobutyric acid

GAD: glutamic acid decarboxylase

GGE: genetic generalized epilepsy

Glut1DS: glucose transporter 1 deficiency syndrome

GTCA: generalized tonic-clonic seizures alone

GTCS: generalized tonic-clonic seizure(s)

HIV: human immunodeficiency virus

ID: intellectual disability

IESS: infantile epileptic spasms syndrome

IGE: idiopathic generalized epilepsy

ILAE: International League Against Epilepsy

IUD: intrauterine device

JAE: juvenile absence epilepsy

JME: juvenile myoclonic epilepsy

KD: ketogenic diet

LC: locus ceruleus

LGS: Lennox–Gastaut syndrome

MCT: medium chain triglyceride

MRI: magnetic resonance imaging

NTS: nucleus tractus solitarius

OCP: oral contraceptive pill

od: once daily

OSA: obstructive sleep apnea

PET: positron emission tomography

qid: four times daily

RS: Rasmussen syndrome

SE: status epilepticus

SeLECTS: self-limited epilepsy with centrotemporal spikes

SUDEP: sudden unexpected death in epilepsy

tid: three times daily

TSC: tuberous sclerosis complex

ULN: upper limit of normal

VNS: vagus nerve stimulation

Foreword

When children and young people with epilepsy (CYPWE) or their caregivers are asked 'Who do you feel is the most important person in your clinical team?' they will invariably answer with the first name of their Epilepsy Specialist Nurse (ESN). At the frontline of epilepsy care, ESNs are the first responders in epilepsy management and patient care, dealing rapidly, calmly, and authoritatively with the multitude of clinical, social, and emotional problems facing CYPWE and their families. So, who better to author a book in the *Fast Facts* series on Epilepsy in Children and Young People. Nicola, Kathryn, Phil and Sheila share their vast experience, distilling it into this concise, focused, and timely publication.

The philosophy is clear throughout: present a balanced and practical overview of diagnosis and management. Chapters cover all aspects of care from seizure types, syndromes, and epidemiology to investigations and management, with tables presenting key points and definitions. The recent classification of epilepsy syndromes is presented in a clear and concise manner, explaining how accurate diagnosis can guide management.

The chapters on pharmacological and non-pharmacological management provide excellent comprehensive guides to the many treatment options available alongside advice that reflects the authors' personal experience. The impact of comorbidities and complications on brain health is emphasized throughout the text, making the point that epilepsy is not just about the seizures.

All of us caring for CYPWE hope that the next decade will bring increasing attention, resources, and improvements to epilepsy care, as health services implement the recommendations of the World Health Organization's *Intersectoral Global Action Plan for Epilepsy and Other Neurological Disorders*. This *Fast Facts* title will support healthcare professionals worldwide in this task.

Sameer M Zuberi

Consultant Paediatric Neurologist and Honorary Professor
Royal Hospital for Children & University of Glasgow
Glasgow, UK

Introduction

Epilepsy is the most common neurological condition in children and young people. Indeed, epilepsy is more likely to begin in childhood, with approximately 50–60% of cases remitting before the young person enters adult services.[1] The seizures experienced by children and young people with epilepsy (CYPWE) are caused by abnormal electrical (neuronal) discharges within the brain. They can be focal or generalized in nature and have a wide range of underlying etiologies and pathologies. Comorbid conditions can occur as a result of seizures or the effects of antiseizure medications (ASM), or epilepsy may be a symptom of, for example, a genetic condition.

Advances in genetic testing have enabled the causes of seizures to be identified more frequently, leading to more precise ASM prescribing. Surgical and non-surgical treatment options are also important in the management of CYPWE.

This concise resource focuses on the investigation, diagnosis, treatment, and management of epilepsy in children and young people, and discusses the transition through to adult services if this is required. Functional (dissociative) seizures (also known as non-epileptic attack disorder or psychogenic non-epileptic seizures) are also discussed as they may be misdiagnosed as epilepsy in children and young people.

We hope that this book will inform all members of the multidisciplinary team involved with the care of CYPWE, as well as parents, caregivers, and education and social care professionals on all aspects of this condition.

References

1. Camfield PR, Camfield CS. What happens to children with epilepsy when they become adults? Some facts and opinions. *Pediatr Neurol* 2014;51:17–23.

Neurology and Neuroscience

1 Seizure types and epidemiology

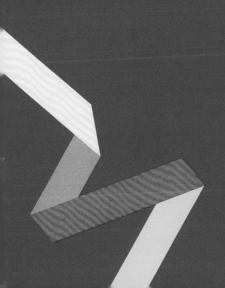

HEALTHCARE

Epilepsy is not a single disease but a heterogeneous group of conditions with a wide range of underlying etiologies and pathologies characterized by recurrent, usually unprovoked, seizures. A seizure is a symptom and represents the clinical manifestation of an abnormal and excessive synchronized discharge of a set of cortical neurons in the brain. Establishing the type(s) of seizure has important implications for:

- choice of investigations
- selection of antiseizure medication (ASM)
- likelihood of an underlying cerebral lesion
- prognosis
- possible genetic transmission.

Seizure types

Depending on the pattern of neuronal involvement (focal, generalized, or unknown onset), the clinical features of a seizure consist of a wide range of sudden and transitory abnormal phenomena, which may include alterations of consciousness, or a motor, sensory, autonomic, or cognitive event (Figure 1.1).

Focal seizures originate from one hemisphere in the brain – the frontal, temporal, parietal, or occipital lobes (Figure 1.2). The child or young person with epilepsy retains awareness during focal aware seizures but does not during focal impaired-awareness seizures. It is essential to identify individuals whose safety may be compromised by loss of awareness during their seizures.

Focal seizures can also be grouped according to their clinical manifestations, such as focal motor and non-motor onset. They can spread rapidly to other cortical areas through neuronal networks, resulting in focal to bilateral tonic-clonic seizures (Figure 1.3). The first symptom of a focal seizure, sometimes called an aura, is vitally important for localizing and lateralizing the epileptogenic focus.

Focal aware seizures. The signs and symptoms of focal aware seizures depend on the site of origin of the abnormal electrical discharges. For example, those arising from the motor cortex can cause automatisms, atonic or clonic seizures, epileptic spasms, and hyperkinetic (agitated thrashing or leg pedaling) movements, or unilateral clonic movements.

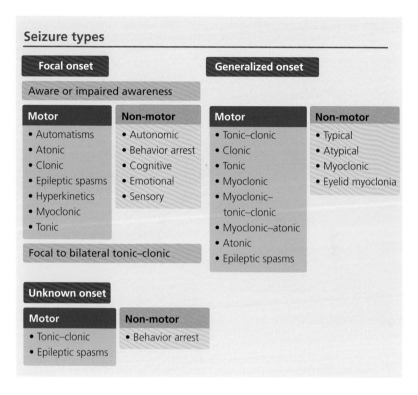

Figure 1.1 Summary of seizure types.

Seizures arising from non-motor regions may produce autonomic, emotional, sensory, cognitive, or behavioral symptoms.

Focal impaired-awareness seizures result in a complete loss or reduction of awareness. Seizures typically last 1–4 minutes. During that time the child or young person may appear awake but becomes unaware of their surroundings; they do not respond normally to instructions or questions. They usually stare and either remain motionless or exhibit impaired function, engaging in repetitive semi-purposeful behavior called automatisms, including chewing, lip smacking, hand wringing, picking, and swallowing. After the seizure they are often sleepy and confused and complain of a headache. This postictal state can last from minutes to hours.

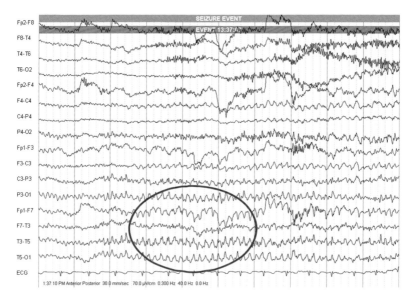

Figure 1.2 EEG showing a focal seizure over the left temporal area (circled).

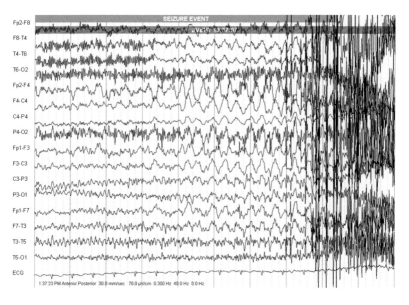

Figure 1.3 EEG showing a bilateral tonic-clonic seizure following from the focal-onset seizure in Figure 1.2.

Focal to generalized bilateral tonic-clonic seizures. Both focal aware and focal impaired-awareness seizures can lead to bilateral tonic-clonic seizures, with bilateral stiffening followed by jerking movements, sometimes with lateral tongue or mouth biting and/or urinary incontinence. The typical duration is 2–3 minutes with jerking movements slowing, becoming more asynchronous and larger in amplitude as the seizure progresses. When the jerking stops the child or young person will become deeply unresponsive for a short while, usually making strenuous breathing noises. Cyanosis may occur. The individual may exhibit postictal impaired awareness and appear confused. Keeping this sequence of events in mind is very important when differentiating between focal-onset seizures and functional (non-epileptic) seizures (see Chapter 10).

Generalized-onset seizures are characterized by widespread involvement of bilateral cortical regions at the outset and are usually accompanied by impaired consciousness. The familiar tonic-clonic seizure often starts with a cry. The individual suddenly falls to the ground and exhibits typical bilateral stiffening (tonic) followed by jerking (clonic) movements, sometimes with lateral tongue or mouth biting and/or urinary incontinence. The absence of an aura helps to delineate these from focal-onset bilateral tonic-clonic seizures, though they may be preceded by a series of myoclonic jerks or absences in some generalized epilepsy syndromes. However, it is important to note that not all focal seizures have an aura, and some auras may be so brief that they are unnoticed by the patient. Therefore, the absence of aura can be regarded as helpful in this context, but not an absolute rule.

Other types of generalized-onset motor seizures include tonic, clonic, myoclonic, myoclonic-tonic-clonic, myoclonic-atonic, atonic, and epileptic spasms. Generalized-onset non-motor seizures include typical and atypical absence seizures and eyelid myoclonia.

Absence seizures usually start in childhood, with the age of onset determining the likelihood of later seizure freedom: for example, 80% of those diagnosed with childhood absence epilepsy (CAE) become seizure free in adolescence.[1] Absences can occur in syndromes that start in adolescence or even early adulthood, such as juvenile myoclonic epilepsy (JME), but this is the exception rather than the rule.

Typical absence seizures usually last 5–10 seconds. They manifest as sudden onset of staring and impaired consciousness, with or without eye blinking and lip smacking. The EEG typically shows a 3-Hz spike-and-wave pattern (Figure 1.4). There is a strong genetic component.

Atypical absence seizures usually begin before 5 years of age in conjunction with other generalized seizure types and learning disability. They last longer than typical absence seizures and are often associated with changes in muscle tone.

Myoclonic seizures consist of sudden brief muscle contractions, either singly or in clusters, that can affect any muscle group.

Clonic seizures are characterized by rhythmic or semi-rhythmic muscle contractions, typically involving the upper extremities, neck, and face.

Tonic seizures cause sudden stiffening of the extensor muscles and are often associated with impaired consciousness and falling to the ground.

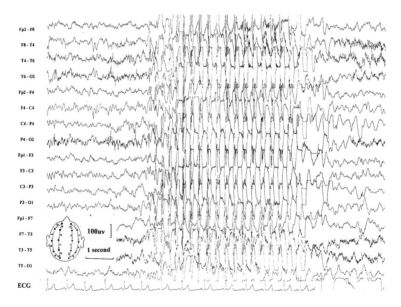

Figure 1.4 EEG showing the 3-Hz spike-and-wave pattern of a typical absence seizure, with characteristic abrupt onset and cessation.

Atonic seizures (also called drop attacks) produce sudden loss of muscle tone with instantaneous collapse (imagine a marionette puppet having its strings cut), often resulting in facial or other injuries.

Epilepsy syndromes

Epilepsy syndromes are defined by characteristic clusters of clinical and EEG features, often supported by specific structural, genetic, metabolic, immune, or infectious etiologic findings (see Chapter 3).

Epidemiology

Incidence and prevalence. Epilepsy is the most common, serious, neurological condition in childhood, affecting between 0.5% and 1% of children around the world.[2] Some data suggest that the incidence of epilepsy may be declining in high-income countries, but a report in 2017 showed that a large cohort in Norway had a cumulative incidence of 0.66% at 10 years of age.[3]

The incidence of epilepsy in children is 41–187 cases per 100 000 persons per year, with the highest incidence in the first year of life, declining to the level observed in adults by the end of the first decade.[4] Prevalence is higher than incidence, with 3.2–6.3 cases per 1000 children reported to have epilepsy in developed countries and 3.6–44 cases per 1000 children in underdeveloped countries.[4] In a study in Scotland in 2021, an estimated 1 in 418 children developed epilepsy before their third birthday. One-third of these developed drug-resistant epilepsy and half had global developmental delay. Etiology was identified in 54% of those diagnosed with epilepsy.[5]

In recent years, there has been a fall in the number of children and young people with epilepsy (CYPWE) but a sharp rise in epilepsy in the elderly, which has now become the most common time in life to develop the condition (Figure 1.5).[6]

Socioeconomic costs. Epilepsy carries a significant socioeconomic burden. A study in Germany evaluating the financial impact of childhood epilepsy highlighted both direct and indirect care costs. Direct costs resulted from frequent hospitalization due to status epilepticus (SE), and the cost of ASM and ancillary treatments. Factors that increased these costs included younger age, the symptomatic cause of the epilepsy, and ASM polytherapy. Indirect costs included

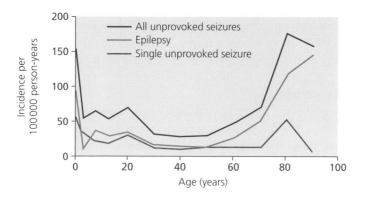

Figure 1.5 Incidence of single unprovoked seizures, epilepsy, and all unprovoked seizures in Iceland between December 1995 and February 1999. Age-specific incidence of all unprovoked seizures was highest in the first year of life (130 cases per 100000 person-years) and in those over 65 years old (110.5 cases per 100000 person-years). Reproduced from Olafsson et al. 2005, with permission from Elsevier.[6]

parents having to reduce their working hours or give up their jobs to care for their child (17% of mothers versus 0.6% of fathers). Indirect costs increased with younger age, longer epilepsy duration, disability, and parental depression.[7] In addition, older children with epilepsy are more likely to have lower attainment at school and be unemployed upon leaving school.

Mortality. Accidents, drowning, burns, aspiration, pneumonia, and SE all confer much higher risks for CYPWE than for the general population. However, many risk factors associated with epilepsy mortality are known to be modifiable.[8,9] The importance of communicating these risks to people with epilepsy has been well evidenced[10,11] and shown to help with risk reduction.[12] Not taking steps to address epilepsy mortality risks can lead to premature deaths in people who are often young and otherwise healthy – it also leaves bereaved families deeply traumatized and often requiring ongoing specialist support.

Sudden unexpected death in epilepsy (SUDEP) is defined as sudden, unexpected, witnessed or unwitnessed, non-traumatic, and non-drowning death that occurs in benign circumstances in an individual with epilepsy, with or without evidence for a seizure and excluding documented SE (seizure duration ≥ 30 minutes or seizures without recovery in between); postmortem examination does not reveal a toxicologic or anatomic cause of death. SUDEP can be further classified, depending on whether a postmortem examination confirmed the diagnosis, whether comorbid conditions contributed to death, and whether the patient was successfully resuscitated after the event (Table 1.1).[13]

In CYPWE, SUDEP accounts for 0.22–6 cases per 1000 person-years.[14] Risk factors for SUDEP in CYPWE are shown in Table 1.2.[15]

TABLE 1.1

Sudden unexpected death in epilepsy definition and classification

Category	Definition
Definite SUDEP	Meets full definition of SUDEP (see text), with confirmation by postmortem examination
Definite SUDEP plus	Meets full definition of SUDEP (see text), but comorbid condition contributes to death
Probable SUDEP	Meets full definition of SUDEP (see text), but no postmortem examination is performed
Probable SUDEP plus	Meets full definition of SUDEP (see text), but comorbid condition contributes to death and no postmortem examination is performed
Possible SUDEP	Death could have been due to SUDEP or other cause
Near-SUDEP	Successful resuscitation after SUDEP event
Near-SUDEP plus	Successful resuscitation after SUDEP event, with other contributing cause

SUDEP, sudden unexpected death in epilepsy.

TABLE 1.2

Risk factors for sudden unexpected death in epilepsy

- History of more than three generalized tonic-clonic seizures per year
- Onset of epilepsy in childhood or adolescence
- Symptomatic epilepsy
- Nocturnal seizures
- Intellectual impairment
- Developmental delay
- Polytherapy
- Treatment-resistant epilepsy
- Subtherapeutic drug concentrations
- Patients not actively being treated for their epilepsy
- Genetic conditions

Adapted from Wicker and Cole 2021.[15]

Generalized tonic-clonic seizures (GTCS), with or without focal onset, are the biggest single risk factor. Risks previously thought to be associated with SUDEP, which later studies suggest are less relevant, include generalized epilepsies (no significant difference compared with focal epilepsies when GTCS are removed), educational level, and mental health disorders. The presence of multiple risks increases mortality exponentially.[16]

People with intellectual disability. In the UK, the Learning Disability Mortality Review (LeDeR) program, which undertakes a root cause analysis for all reported deaths of people with intellectual disability (ID), reported epilepsy and SE as being among the five most common causes of death in 4- to 17-year-olds between 2018 and 2021, and epilepsy was the most common long-term health condition associated with an earlier age at death.[17]

In a literature search between 1990 and 2014, 16 studies were identified (in the USA, UK, Finland, Netherlands, Sweden, Denmark, and Japan) in which concomitant epilepsy in people with ID increased the risk of death, particularly in those who had experienced recent seizures.[18]

In New South Wales, Australia, a retrospective study of people hospitalized with an epilepsy diagnosis between 2005 and 2015 showed that CYPWE with ID had a higher mortality risk than those with epilepsy alone. The risk of death increased with specific comorbidities, especially neurological and respiratory disorders.[19]

Pregnancy. Women with epilepsy who are pregnant (or have recently given birth) are also a vulnerable group. A national enquiry by MBRRACE-UK (Mothers and Babies: Reducing Risk through Audits and Confidential Enquiries across the UK) in 2020 flagged a doubling of SUDEP among this group between 2016 and 2018.[20]

In a retrospective cohort study of pregnant women in 2007–2011 in the USA, women with epilepsy were found to have a significantly higher risk of death than those without epilepsy (80 vs 6 deaths during hospital deliveries per 100000 pregnancies).[21] Likewise, in Denmark, maternal mortality was found to be more than five times higher in women with epilepsy than in those without epilepsy (41.7 vs 8.2 deaths per 100000 pregnancies).[22]

Although these studies analyzed data from women of all ages, it is important that pregnant teenage girls should also receive counseling regarding the high risk.

Key points – seizure types and epidemiology

- Epilepsy is a heterogeneous group of conditions with a wide range of underlying etiologies and pathologies characterized by recurrent, usually unprovoked, seizures.
- A seizure manifests as an abnormal and excessive synchronized discharge of a set of cortical neurons in the brain, which can result in alterations of consciousness, or a motor, sensory, autonomic, or cognitive event.
- Seizures can be focal, generalized, or of unknown onset.
- Epilepsy is one of the most common chronic neurological conditions in childhood. The highest incidence occurs in the first year of life, and prevalence is highest in underdeveloped countries.
- The socioeconomic cost of epilepsy in children and adolescents is significant. Direct costs include ASM and frequent hospitalization, while indirect costs include the time parents need to take off work to care for their children.
- There are many risk factors associated with epilepsy mortality in CYPWE, including accidents, drowning, burns, aspiration, pneumonia, SUDEP, and SE. Many of these are preventable, and communicating the risks helps to reduce the number of deaths.
- Young people with ID and teenage girls who are pregnant (or who have recently given birth) have an increased mortality risk.

References

1. National Institute for Health and Care Excellence (NICE). *Clinical Knowledge Summaries (CKS). Epilepsy: What is the prognosis?* NICE, 2023. cks.nice.org.uk/topics/epilepsy/background-information/prognosis, last accessed 1 November 2023.

2. Olusanya B, Wright SM, Nair MKC et al. Global burden of childhood epilepsy, intellectual disability, and sensory impairments. *Pediatrics* 2020;146:e20192623.

3. Aaberg KM, Gunnes N, Bakken IJ et al. Incidence and prevalence of childhood epilepsy: a nationwide cohort study. *Pediatrics* 2017;139:e20163908.

4. Camfield P, Camfield C. Incidence, prevalence and aetiology of seizures and epilepsy in children. *Epileptic Disord* 2015;17:117–23.

5. Symonds JD, Elliott KS, Shetty J et al. Early childhood epilepsies: epidemiology, classification, aetiology, and socio-economic determinants. *Brain* 2021;144:2879–91.

6. Olafsson E, Ludvigsson P, Hesdorffer D et al. Incidence of unprovoked seizures and epilepsy in Iceland and assessment of the epilepsy syndrome classification: a prospective study. *Lancet Neurol* 2005;4:627–34.

7. Riechmann J, Strzelczyk A, Reese JP et al. Costs of epilepsy and cost-driving factors in children, adolescents, and their caregivers in Germany. *Epilepsia* 2015;56:1388–97.

8. Shankar R, Jalihal V, Walker M et al. A community study in Cornwall UK of sudden unexpected death in epilepsy (SUDEP) in a 9-year population sample. *Seizure* 2014;23:382–5.

9. McCabe J, McLean B, Henley W et al. Sudden unexpected death in epilepsy (SUDEP) and seizure safety: modifiable and non-modifiable risk factors differences between primary and secondary care. *Epilepsy Behav* 2021;115:107637.

10. Smart C, Page G, Shankar R, Newman C. Keep safe: the when, why and how of epilepsy risk communication. *Seizure* 2020;78:136–49.

11. Waddell B, McColl K, Turner C et al. Are we discussing SUDEP? A retrospective case note analysis. *Seizure* 2013;22:74–6.

12. Shankar R, Henley W, Boland C et al. Decreasing the risk of sudden unexpected death in epilepsy: structure communication of risk factors for premature mortality in people with epilepsy. *Eur J Neurol* 2018;25:1121–7.

13. Nashef L, So EL, Ryvlin P, Tomson T. Unifying the definitions of sudden unexpected death in epilepsy. *Epilepsia* 2012;53:227–33.

14. Abdel-Mannan O, Venkatesan TC, Sutcliffe AG. Paediatric sudden unexpected death in epilepsy (SUDEP): is it truly unexplained? *Paediatr Child Health* 2022;32:382–7.

15. Wicker E, Cole JW. Sudden unexpected death in epilepsy (SUDEP): a review of risk factors and possible interventions in children. *J Pediatr Pharmacol Ther* 2021;26:556–64.

16. Abdel-Mannan O, Taylor H, Donner EJ, Sutcliffe AG. A systematic review of sudden unexpected death in epilepsy (SUDEP) in childhood. *Epilepsy Behav* 2019;90:99–106.

17. White A, Sheehan R, Ding J et al. *Learning from Lives and Deaths – People with a learning disability and autistic people (LeDeR) report for 2021 (LeDeR Annual Report 2021)*. Autism and learning disability partnership, King's College, London, 2021. kcl.ac.uk/research/leder, last accessed 15 November 2022.

18. Robertson J, Hatton C, Emerson E, Baines S. Mortality in people with intellectual disabilities and epilepsy: a systematic review. *Seizure* 2015;29:123–33.

19. Liao P, Vajdic CM, Reppermund S et al. Mortality rate, risk factors, and causes of death in people with epilepsy and intellectual disability. *Seizure* 2022;101:75–82.

20. Knight M, Bunch K, Patel R (eds) et al. *Saving Lives, Improving Mothers' Care. Lessons learned to inform maternity care from the UK and Ireland confidential enquiries into maternal deaths and morbidity 2018-20*. MBRRACE-UK, 2022. npeu.ox.ac.uk/assets/downloads/mbrrace-uk/reports/maternal-report-2022/MBRRACE-UK_Maternal_MAIN_Report_2022_UPDATE.pdf, last accessed 1 November 2023.

21. MacDonald SC, Bateman BT, McElrath TF, Hernandez-Diaz S. Mortality and morbidity during delivery hospitalization among pregnant women with epilepsy in the United States. *JAMA Neurol* 2015;72:981–8.

22. Christensen J, Vestergaard C, Bech BH. Maternal death in women with epilepsy: smaller scope studies. *Neurology* 2018; 91:e1716–20.

Neurology and
Neuroscience

2 Classification and prognosis

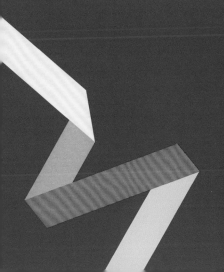

HEALTHCARE

Classification

The Nosology and Definitions Task Force of the International League Against Epilepsy (ILAE) has published four position papers that define and classify epilepsy syndromes at various ages through childhood and adolescence.[1-4] We highly recommend reading these papers for full descriptions of the clinical course and EEG features of each epilepsy syndrome, along with their differential diagnoses. In this chapter, we discuss some of the syndromes more commonly seen in children and young people with epilepsy (CYPWE) in clinical practice.

Epilepsy syndromes are defined by groups of characteristic clinical features related to age at seizure onset, family history of epilepsy, seizure type(s), and neurological signs and symptoms, aided by appropriate investigations, including EEG and brain imaging. The ILAE primarily categorizes epilepsy syndromes in children and young people by age of onset: in neonates or infants (<2 years old), in children (2–12 years old), or at a variable age, including the idiopathic generalized epilepsies (IGE), which have an onset in childhood or adolescence (Table 2.1).

Epilepsy syndromes can be focal or generalized in nature, with generalized epilepsy syndromes classified as genetic generalized epilepsy (GGE) syndromes. IGE syndromes form a subgroup of GGE to differentiate these common epilepsies from the rarer GGE syndromes.[4]

Diagnosing an epileptic syndrome enables clinicians to define the likely prognosis, provide reasonable genetic counseling, and choose the most appropriate antiseizure medication (ASM). Most epilepsy syndromes start in childhood and continue into adulthood.

Epilepsy syndromes with onset in neonates and infants

The ILAE divides epilepsy syndromes in children under 2 years old into two main groups: self-limited epilepsy syndromes and developmental and/or epileptic encephalopathies (DEE). There are also several etiology-specific syndromes in this age group.[1]

Self-limited epilepsy syndromes. The term 'benign', which does not take into consideration the comorbidities that some individuals have, has been replaced with the term 'self-limited'. Seizures tend to be responsive to ASM and, as the term 'self-limited' suggests,

TABLE 2.1

Epilepsy syndromes in children and adolescents by age of onset

Epilepsy syndrome	Formerly known as
Neonatal/infantile (<2 years)	
• Self-limited epilepsy syndromes	
– Self-limited (non-familial or familial) neonatal epilepsy (SeLNE, SeLFNE)	Benign familial neonatal seizures
– Self-limited familial neonatal-infantile epilepsy (SeLFNIE)	Benign (non-familial or familial) infantile seizures
– Self-limited (non-familial or familial) infantile epilepsy (SeLIE, SeLFIE)	
– Genetic epilepsy with febrile seizures plus (GEFS+)	
– Myoclonic epilepsy in infancy (MEI)	
• Developmental and/or epileptic encephalopathies (DEE)	
– Early infantile DEE (EIDEE)	Ohtahara syndrome and early myoclonic encephalopathy
– Epilepsy in infancy with migrating focal seizures (EIMFS)	
– Infantile epileptic spasms syndrome (IESS)	West syndrome and infantile spasms
– Dravet syndrome (DS)	Severe myoclonic epilepsy of infancy
• Etiology-specific syndromes	
– *KCNQ2*-DEE	
– Pyridoxine-dependent (*ALDH7A1*)-DEE (PD-DEE)	
– Pyridox(am)ine 5'-phosphate deficiency (PNPO)-DEE (P5PD-DEE)	
– *CDKL5*-DEE	
– *PCDH19* clustering epilepsy	
– Glucose transporter 1 deficiency syndrome (Glut1DS)	
– Sturge–Weber syndrome (SWS)	
– Gelastic seizures with hypothalamic hamartoma (GS-HH)	

CONTINUED

TABLE 2.1 CONTINUED

Epilepsy syndromes in children and adolescents by age of onset

Epilepsy syndrome	Formerly known as
Childhood (2–12 years)	
• Self-limited focal epilepsies	
– Self-limited epilepsy with centrotemporal spikes (SeLECTS)	(benign) Rolandic epilepsy, (benign/childhood) epilepsy with centrotemporal spikes
– Self-limited epilepsy with autonomic seizures (SeLEAS)	Panayiotopoulos syndrome, early-onset (benign) occipital epilepsy
– Childhood occipital visual epilepsy (COVE)*	Late-onset (benign) occipital epilepsy, idiopathic childhood occipital epilepsy (Gastaut type)
– Photosensitive occipital lobe epilepsy (POLE)*	Idiopathic photosensitive occipital lobe epilepsy
• Genetic generalized epilepsies	
– Childhood absence epilepsy (CAE)	Pyknolepsy, petit mal
– Epilepsy with myoclonic absence (EMA)	Bureau and Tassinari syndrome
– Epilepsy with eyelid myoclonia (EEM)	Jeavons syndrome
• Developmental and/or epileptic encephalopathies	
– Epilepsy with myoclonic–atonic seizures (EMatS)	Doose syndrome
– Lennox–Gastaut syndrome (LGS)	
– DEE with spike-and-wave activation in sleep (DEE-SWAS)	Epileptic encephalopathy with continuous spike-and-wave in sleep, atypical (benign) partial epilepsy (pseudo-Lennox syndrome)
– Epileptic encephalopathy with spike-and-wave activation in sleep (EE-SWAS)	

CONTINUED

TABLE 2.1 CONTINUED
– Hemiconvulsion-hemiplegia-
epilepsy syndrome

– Febrile infection-related epilepsy syndrome (FIRES)	Acute encephalitis with refractory, repetitive partial seizures, devastating epileptic encephalopathy in school-aged children

Variable age (≤18 or ≥19 years)

• Generalized epilepsy syndromes
  – Juvenile absence epilepsy (JAE)
  – Juvenile myoclonic epilepsy (JME)
  – Epilepsy with generalized tonic-clonic seizures alone (GTCA)

• Focal epilepsy syndromes with genetic, structural, or genetic-structural etiologies

– Familial mesial temporal lobe epilepsy (FMTLE)	Autosomal dominant lateral temporal lobe epilepsy

  – Epilepsy with auditory features (EAF)
  – Sleep-related hypermotor (hyperkinetic) epilepsy (SHE)

– Familial focal epilepsy with variable foci (FFEVF)	Familial partial epilepsy with variable foci, autosomal dominant partial epilepsy with variable foci

• Combined generalized and focal epilepsy syndromes with polygenic etiology
  – Epilepsy with reading-induced seizures (EwRIS)

CONTINUED

TABLE 2.1 CONTINUED

Epilepsy syndromes in children and adolescents by age of onset

Epilepsy syndrome	Formerly known as
Variable age (≤ 18 or ≥ 19 years) *continued*	
• Epilepsy syndromes with DEE or progressive neurological deterioration	
– Progressive myoclonus epilepsies (PME)	
– Febrile infection-related epilepsy syndrome (FIRES)	
• Etiology-specific syndromes	
– Mesial temporal lobe epilepsy with hippocampal sclerosis (MTLE-HS)	
– Rasmussen syndrome (RS)	Rasmussen encephalitis

*Also classified as occurring at any age (≤ 18 or ≥ 19 years).
DEE, developmental and/or epileptic encephalopathy.

spontaneous remission is likely. Children with these epilepsies tend to have normal cognition or mild cognitive impairment only.

Developmental and/or epileptic encephalopathies can be further divided by age of onset into early infantile DEE (EIDEE), which occurs in infants under 3 months old, and other DEE that can occur at any time during the early or late infantile period. The neurodevelopmental impairment typically seen in children with DEE may be due to the underlying etiology and/or the adverse effects of uncontrolled seizures.

Infantile epileptic spasms syndrome (IESS) encompasses all cases of infantile spasms, including West syndrome, which is characterized by epileptic spasms, hypsarrhythmia, and developmental delay or regression. Previously, epileptic spasms could not be diagnosed unless this triad of symptoms was present. However, infants with IESS often lack one of the criteria, which could lead to delayed diagnosis and treatment. Prompt treatment is associated with better outcomes, hence the wider classification of IESS, with the term West syndrome reserved for children with all three symptoms.

IESS is a serious but rare type of epilepsy that affects 30 per 100 000 liveborn infants. It is characterized by sudden brief tonic contractions of axial muscles (flexor, extensor, or mixed). The spasms often occur in frequent clusters throughout the day. IESS has onset at 1–24 months of age (peaking at 3–12 months). A background EEG most typically shows hypsarrhythmia and multifocal or focal epileptiform discharges.[1]

Prognosis. IESS carries a high lifetime mortality rate. For those who survive, 75% have intellectual disability (ID) and more than 50% have seizures that continue into childhood and adult life. Treatment can be extremely difficult. Initially this generally involves the use of corticosteroids with or without vigabatrin. Prognosis is more favorable for infants with preceding normal development, no known cause, and prompt initiation of syndrome-specific treatment.[1]

Dravet syndrome is a rare genetic form of childhood epilepsy affecting about 6 per 100 000 live births. Seizures usually manifest at 3–9 months of age (range 1–20 months). They can be afebrile or febrile and are most commonly hemiclonic focal seizures, which can alternate left and right from seizure to seizure, or focal to bilateral tonic-clonic and/or generalized tonic-clonic. Seizures are often prolonged, lasting over 10 minutes. Other seizure types, including myoclonic and atypical absence, usually appear between the ages of 1 and 4 years. Seizures can be very difficult to control and often develop into convulsive and non-convulsive status epilepticus (SE). By the age of 14–16 years, seizures become less frequent, but still occur. Photosensitivity can develop, more commonly in younger children and less commonly after the age of 5 years.[1]

Prognosis. Initial early child development is normal, but it starts to slow down and children lose skills, in particular speech and language, from the second year of life. Ataxia develops and gait can also be affected. The EEG is normal or slow early in the condition but soon becomes abnormal, showing focal, multifocal, and generalized discharges after the age of 2 years. MRI brain scans are usually normal at seizure onset. Mild cerebral and cerebellar atrophy may evolve later, with a minority of children having hippocampal sclerosis, although surgery is not indicated. Sadly, there is a higher incidence of sudden unexpected death in epilepsy (SUDEP) in children with Dravet syndrome under 5 years old.

Etiology-specific syndromes is an emerging class of epilepsy syndromes in neonates and infants in which a distinct electroclinical phenotype has a strong association with a specific genetic, structural, metabolic, immune, or infectious etiology (see Table 2.1). Most etiology-specific syndromes in children under 2 years old are DEE. It is likely that further etiology-specific syndromes will be added to this class over time.

Epilepsy syndromes with onset in childhood

The ILAE divides epilepsy syndromes in children aged 2–12 years into three main groups: self-limited focal epilepsies, GGE, and DEE which often have both focal and generalized seizures.[2] Childhood absence epilepsy (CAE), an IGE, also typically starts during childhood.

Some childhood epilepsy syndromes may have evolved from neonatal or infantile epilepsies: for example, IESS can evolve into Lennox-Gastaut syndrome.

Self-limited focal epilepsies, which have previously been termed 'benign' or 'idiopathic', usually have an unknown etiology. However, as many individuals have a positive family history of epilepsy, underlying genetic factors are likely. There are four syndromes in this category, which together make up 25% of childhood epilepsies.[2] Self-limited epilepsy with centrotemporal spikes (SeLECTS) and self-limited epilepsy with autonomic seizures (SeLEAS) usually remit by adolescence, whereas childhood occipital visual epilepsy (COVE) and photosensitive occipital lobe epilepsy (POLE) may persist after adolescence.

Self-limited epilepsy with centrotemporal spikes is one of the most common types of childhood epilepsy, affecting about 6.1 per 100 000 children under 16 years of age per year. It is dominated by nocturnal focal to bilateral tonic-clonic seizures and/or brief focal seizures involving clonic or tonic activity of the throat/tongue and one side of the lower face, with onset usually between 4 and 10 years of age (range 3–14 years). Both sexes are affected, with a slight male predominance (60%). SeLECTS has a typical EEG pattern of high amplitude centrotemporal biphasic epileptiform abnormalities.[2]

Prognosis. Seizures usually remit by puberty, even in those whose seizures were difficult to control, and the social outcome in adults is very good.

Genetic generalized epilepsies. All generalized epilepsy syndromes with onset in childhood, namely CAE, epilepsy with myoclonic absence (EMA), and epilepsy with eyelid myoclonia (EEM), have a genetic (polygenic) etiology. Cognition and neurological examinations, and response to ASM, are variable. It is worth noting that seizures in infants under 2 years old will always have focal onset as there is insufficient neuronal pathway development to support generalized epilepsy.

Childhood absence epilepsy occurs in about 6–8 per 100 000 children per year and accounts for approximately 18% of epilepsy in school-age children. Seizures usually start in children aged 4–10 years (range 2–13 years). They can occur 10–100 times a day, typically lasting 5–15 seconds, with a sudden cessation in activity, sudden loss of awareness, and staring. There may be some facial automatisms. Atypical absences, which last longer than 15 seconds and include frequent automatisms and brief jerks of the head, are important exclusion criteria for CAE, instead suggesting the presence of a DEE.[4]

Prognosis. CAE usually responds to medication, and remits by early adolescence in 80% of patients.[5] The remainder may evolve into other IGE syndromes. Children and young people with CAE develop normally but frequent absences can cause some learning difficulties, often due to missed schooling. Memory and concentration may also be affected.[4]

Developmental and/or epileptic encephalopathies include syndromes in which the underlying cause (developmental encephalopathy) or the epileptic activity (epileptic encephalopathy) or both contribute to severe cognitive and behavioral impairments (see Table 2.1).

Lennox-Gastaut syndrome (LGS) usually starts in children aged between 18 months and 8 years (peak age of onset 3–5 years). IESS, early infantile DEE, and epilepsy of infancy with migrating focal seizures often evolve into LGS. Seizure types are mixed and occur multiple times a day. Cognitive impairment is usually present before the onset of seizures and can be associated with behavioral problems.[2]

Prognosis is poor, with drug-resistant epilepsy and mild to profound ID.

Epilepsy syndromes with onset at variable age
There are several important syndromes that can begin at a variable age (≤18 years or ≥19 years). They are divided into GGE syndromes,

self-limited focal epilepsy syndromes, focal epilepsy syndromes with genetic, structural, or genetic-structural etiologies, combined generalized and focal epilepsy syndromes with polygenic etiology, and DEEs and epilepsy syndromes with progressive neurological deterioration (see Table 2.1). Two etiology-specific syndromes have also been described: mesial temporal lobe epilepsy with hippocampal sclerosis and Rasmussen syndrome.[3]

Idiopathic generalized epilepsy syndromes. An estimated 15–20% of all people with epilepsy have an IGE. Those that present at a variable age are juvenile absence epilepsy (JAE), juvenile myoclonic epilepsy (JME), and epilepsy with generalized tonic-clonic seizures alone (GTCA). CAE has an onset in childhood (see above).

Juvenile absence epilepsy is less common than CAE but accounts for 2.4–3.1% of new-onset epilepsy in CYPWE. Onset is usually at 13 years of age (range 8–20 years). It is more common in girls than boys. Absences usually last for 5–20 seconds, with longer atypical absences and prominent myoclonic jerks being important exclusion criteria for the syndrome. Generalized tonic-clonic seizures occur in 8 out of 10 children and young people with JAE. The seizures usually begin shortly after the absences and often mark the point where the epilepsy comes to medical attention and treatment is started.[4]

Prognosis. Children and young people with JAE have a normal intellectual ability, but frequent absences can result in memory and learning impairment.

Juvenile myoclonic epilepsy is a common type of epilepsy, with a prevalence of 1–3 cases per 10000 people, and accounts for about 9.3% of all epilepsies. It usually occurs between the ages of 10 and 24 years (range 8–40 years), with 5–15% of cases evolving from CAE. People with JME have myoclonic jerks (needed for diagnosis), tonic-clonic seizures, and often absences, though these are usually more subtle than those found in JAE. Seizures can occur at any time of day but typically occur within an hour of waking. Just under half of people with JME have photosensitivity. Sleep deprivation, often accompanied by alcohol consumption, is a major seizure trigger in this type of epilepsy.[4]

Prognosis. In general, JME is a lifelong condition, requiring long-term treatment.

Generalized tonic-clonic seizures alone involve the development of generalized tonic-clonic seizures, usually within 2 hours of waking. The presence of any other seizure types is an exclusion criterion. Seizures are often provoked by sleep deprivation. Age of onset is wide (5–40 years), but most seizures start between 10 and 25 years of age. MRI is normal, with EEG showing 3–5.5 Hz generalized spike-and-wave or poly spike-and-wave discharges.[4]

Prognosis. Like JME, GTCA is generally a lifelong condition.

Prognosis

As can be seen in the examples of epilepsy syndromes above, the prognosis of childhood epilepsy is extremely variable and depends on the underlying cause and syndromic diagnosis. However, in general, 50–60% of CYPWE eventually become seizure free following ASM withdrawal, attaining complete remission.[6] The other 40–50% of patients continue to have seizures with varying degrees of frequency and severity. Some have a remitting–relapsing course, fluctuating between periods of seizure freedom and recurrence. A good example of this is mesial temporal lobe epilepsy with hippocampal sclerosis, where patients often achieve seizure freedom following the initiation of ASM but relapse months to years later with a poor response to additional medication.[7]

Identifying which CYPWE will have a poor prognosis is clearly important for planning long-term management and surgery, and when considering lifestyle issues and risk, including that of SUDEP.

Some pediatric epilepsy syndromes, such as CAE or SeLECTS, have an excellent prognosis. Others like JME can, for most people, be considered lifelong conditions, although treatment with ASM is often highly effective. Unfortunately, some pediatric epilepsies have a very poor prognosis. DEE, such as IESS (including West syndrome) and Dravet syndrome, are usually associated with developmental regression, often leading to severe ID, frequent seizures with a poor response to ASM, and a significant mortality rate.

Factors that indicate a poor prognosis for seizure control include:
- poor response to the initial ASM treatment
- symptomatic cause
- high seizure frequency before ASM treatment
- generalized tonic-clonic seizures
- generalized epileptiform activity on the EEG
- family history of epilepsy
- comorbid psychiatric history.

Key points – classification and prognosis

- Epilepsy syndromes in children and young people are primarily classified by age of seizure onset: in neonates or infants under 2 years old, children aged 2–12 years old, or children and young people of variable age, including IGE which have an onset in childhood or adolescence.
- Seizures in neonates always have a focal onset as there is insufficient neuronal pathway development to support generalized epilepsy.
- Childhood-onset epilepsies are a heterogeneous group of conditions with variable prognosis and treatment pathways.
- Many childhood epilepsy syndromes have a genetic component and full genome sequencing should be considered (see Chapter 4).
- Identifying which CYPWE will have a poor prognosis is important for planning long-term management, and when considering lifestyle issues and risks.

References

1. Zuberi SM, Wirrell E, Yozawitz E et al. ILAE classification and definition of epilepsy syndromes with onset in neonates and infants: position statement by the ILAE Task Force on Nosology and Definitions. *Epilepsia* 2022;63:1349–97.

2. Specchio N, Wirrell EC, Scheffer IE et al. International League Against Epilepsy classification and definition of epilepsy syndromes with onset in childhood: position paper by the ILAE Task Force on Nosology and Definitions. *Epilepsia* 2022;63:1398–442.

3. Riney K, Bogacz A, Somerville E et al. International League Against Epilepsy classification and definition of epilepsy syndromes with onset at a variable age: position paper by the ILAE Task Force on Nosology and Definitions. *Epilepsia* 2022;63:1443–74.

4. Hirsch E, French J, Scheffer IE et al. ILAE definition of the idiopathic generalized epilepsy syndromes: position paper by the ILAE Task Force on Nosology and Definitions. *Epilepsia* 2022;63:1475–99.

5. National Institute for Health and Care Excellence. *Clinical Knowledge Summaries (CKS). Epilepsy: What is the prognosis?* NICE, 2023. cks.nice.org.uk/topics/epilepsy/background-information/prognosis, last accessed 1 November 2023.

6. Camfield PR, Camfield CS. What happens to children with epilepsy when they become adults? Some facts and opinions. *Pediatr Neurol* 2014;51:17–23.

7. Berg AT. The natural history of mesial temporal lobe epilepsy. *Curr Opin Neurol* 2008;21:173–8.

**Neurology and
Neuroscience**

3 Causes and triggers

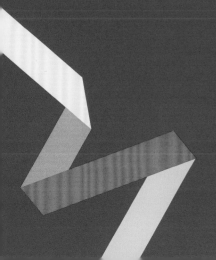

HEALTHCARE

Epilepsies in children and young people have a wide range of etiologies. There is also considerable overlap, with some syndromes having different causes despite sharing common phenotypes. Infantile epileptic spasms syndrome (IESS), for example, may have a genetic cause, or may be due to a structural etiology such as hypoxic injury, cerebrovascular accident, or a neurocutaneous condition.

Genetic causes

As Chapter 2 indicates, genetic etiology is common in childhood epilepsies, and may be attributed to either chromosomal or gene abnormalities. Genetic factors that can lead to epilepsy include:

- inherited gene abnormalities with autosomal dominant, autosomal recessive, or Mendelian inheritance
- acquired gene abnormalities: de novo, sporadic, mosaicism, germline, or somatic
- polygenic/complex genetic etiology.

Well-replicated genetics, derived from appropriately designed family studies, have become the basis of diagnostic testing (see Genetic testing, page 62).

Chromosomal abnormalities. A wide range of chromosomal abnormalities are associated with epilepsy. Some can be recognized by the patient's seizure type and EEG features. Inevitably, they are associated with other symptoms, usually intellectual disability (ID) and dysmorphic facial features, and sometimes abnormalities of other organs or limbs. Some, such as Down syndrome, give rise to an increased incidence of epilepsy without it being inevitable (around 10% in childhood but with a second peak after the third decade of life when late-onset myoclonic epilepsy, which is associated with the early onset of Alzheimer-type dementia, affects 50%).[1]

The severity of epilepsy and the types of seizures experienced can be extremely variable. Some chromosomal abnormalities are associated with a much higher incidence of epilepsy. For example, Ring chromosome 14 syndrome is a rare disorder that always causes epilepsy. Seizures are intractable, and ID, microcephaly, facial dysmorphism, and cardiac and ocular abnormalities are present.[2] 15q13.3 microdeletion syndrome also causes epilepsy in around 30% of cases. Typically, this presents as a genetic generalized epilepsy with most patients experiencing absences. Other generalized seizures also occur and most children will experience at least two different seizure types; one-third will present with focal, impaired-awareness, non-motor-onset seizures.[3]

Recently, it has been shown that different genetic abnormalities can give rise to the same phenotype. For example, a child or young person with juvenile myoclonic epilepsy (JME) may have a genetic mutation at several locations. Recurrent microdeletions at 15q13.3, 15q11.2, and 16p13.22, are all susceptibility alleles for JME. The current thinking is that susceptibility alleles have a variant that contributes to the epilepsy but is not the sole cause of the condition.[4]

Gene abnormalities. Table 3.1 gives examples of gene abnormalities identified in certain epilepsy syndromes. Around 34% of genetic changes have been identified in genes encoding ion channels. Mutations in *SCN1A* and *SCN2A* alter ion channel function, which affects the transmission of depolarizing impulses in brain networks. *KCNQ2* mutations encode for voltage-gated potassium channel subunits, which ultimately regulate excitability in central and peripheral neurons.[5] Sometimes, the same mutation is found in different epilepsy syndromes: for example, variants in the *GABRG2* gene have been linked to childhood absence epilepsy (CAE), genetic epilepsy with febrile seizures plus (GEFS+), and JME.

Structural causes

There are numerous structural causes for epilepsy. The most common involve traumatic brain injury or ischemic/hypoxic injury. These can clearly occur at any age. For most structural epilepsies, high-quality cranial MRI is the investigation of choice, and advances in imaging techniques over the last few decades have led to increased diagnosis and understanding of these etiologies (Figure 3.1).[6–8]

Mesial temporal lobe epilepsy with hippocampal sclerosis (MTLE-HS) is the most common focal epilepsy (see Figure 3.1a). The precise cause of hippocampal sclerosis remains unclear; risk factors include injury due to prolonged febrile convulsions (or other seizure types) and genetic susceptibility. Head trauma, infections, or anoxia can also

TABLE 3.1

Examples of gene abnormalities identified in epilepsy syndromes

Syndrome	Gene	Example of gene product
Self-limited (familial) neonatal epilepsy	KCNQ2, KCNQ3	Voltage-gated potassium channel subunits
Self-limited familial neonatal-infantile epilepsy	SCN2A	Voltage-gated sodium channel subunits, type 2
Sleep-related hypermotor (hyperkinetic) epilepsy	CHRNA4, CHRNA2, CHRNB2, DEPDC5, KCNT1, NPRL2, NPRL3, PRIMA1	Nicotinic acetylcholine receptor subunits
Epilepsy with auditory features	LGI1, RELN, MICAL1	Leucine-rich glioma-inactivated protein
Genetic epilepsy with febrile seizures plus, and Dravet syndrome	SCN1A, SCN1B, SCN2A	Voltage-gated sodium channel subunits
	GABRG2	GABA-A receptor subunits, type 2
Epilepsy of infancy with migrating focal features	SCN1A	Voltage-gated sodium channel subunits, type 1

GABA, γ-aminobutyric acid.

damage the hippocampus. Recent work has suggested the possibility of limbic encephalitis being a more common cause than previously thought, even in people who show no clinical signs.[9]

Focal seizures with or without impaired awareness often begin with a rising sensation from the stomach, feelings of fear or anxiety, a sensation of déjà vu or jamais vu, or an abnormal, generally unpleasant taste or smell. These warnings typically evolve to focal impaired-awareness seizures involving automatisms such as chewing or lip smacking, fiddling with clothes, or twisting movements of the hands. Some of these seizures will evolve into generalized tonic-clonic seizures.

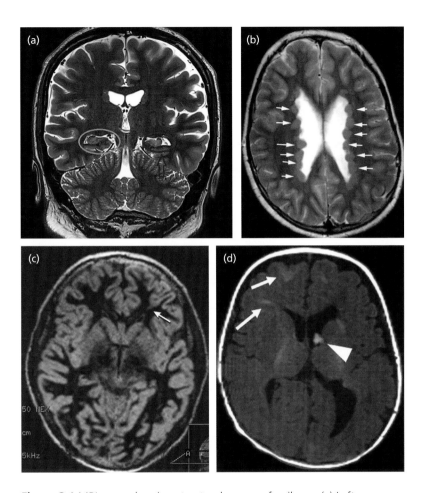

Figure 3.1 MRI scans showing structural causes of epilepsy. (a) Left hippocampal sclerosis (red) in a patient with mesial temporal lobe epilepsy – there is greater volume loss compared with the right hippocampus (blue), reproduced courtesy of Uhomachinky under license CC BY-SA 4.0; (b) bilateral periventricular nodular heterotopia, reproduced from Barkovich 2022, under license CC BY 4.0;[6] (c) Focal cortical dysplasia in a 12-year-old boy who became seizure free 2.5 years after resection, reprinted from Wong-Kisiel et al. 2016, with permission from Elsevier;[7] (d) subependymal nodule (arrowhead) and white matter and cortical lesions (arrows) in a 4-month-old infant with tuberous sclerosis, reproduced from Radhakrishnan and Verma 2011, under license CC BY 4.0.[8]

The condition is often medically intractable, but epilepsy surgery involving resection of part or all of the mesial temporal lobe can render some children and young people with epilepsy (CYPWE) seizure free.

Malformations of cortical development commonly cause seizures in CYPWE. They arise because of an interruption of cellular migration from the periventricular region to the cerebral cortex in early intrauterine life, and several may coexist in the same individual. Genetic or chromosomal abnormalities can contribute to migration abnormalities, as can anoxia or intrauterine infection, although to a lesser extent. Developmental and cognitive outcome may be poor in children who develop epileptic (infantile) spasms or generalized seizures. These are commonly associated with heterotopias, focal cortical dysplasias, and tuberous sclerosis (TS) (see below). For these CYPWE, early optimization of seizure control, perhaps involving surgery, is paramount.[10]

Heterotopias (literally meaning 'out of place') occur when normal neurons migrate to the wrong place due to a malfunction of apoptosis (programmed cell death). Gray matter heterotopia is a malformation where cortical cells (gray matter) line the lateral ventricles (bilateral periventricular nodular heterotopia) (see Figure 3.1b) or appear in subcortical white matter (subcortical nodular heterotopia).[6] Seizures occur in 80–90% of children.[11] Subcortical band heterotopia involves cortical cells failing to migrate to their correct location and forming a band between the lateral ventricular wall and the cortex, usually bilaterally. Seizures may or may not be present, can begin at any age, and correlate with the thickness of the subcortical band. ID is usual, with the severity dictated by the extent of the heterotopia.

Lissencephaly (smooth brain) involves reduced gyration and either cerebral cortical thickening (type I) or a nodular appearance to the cortex (type II). Seizures occur in more than 90% of individuals and usually start in the first year of life.[11] ID is usually severe, and many children have bulbar difficulties, resulting in problematic feeding and respiratory function.

Polymicrogyria involves excessive gyration, abnormal layering, and gyral fusion in the cerebral cortex. It can be associated with

Acardi syndrome and bilateral perisylvian syndrome. The development of epilepsy is common, with around 50% of children developing seizures in the first year of life, around 70% within the first 5 years, and a few in later childhood and adolescence.[11] Rarely, a cleft in the brain, known as schizencephaly, can occur. Polymicrogyria line the cleft which extends from the ependyma of the ventricles to the pia matter.

Focal cortical dysplasia, localized regions of malformed cerebral cortex, is a common cause of focal seizures (see Figure 3.1c). The precise nature of seizures depends on the location and extent of the dysplasia, but they occur in almost all affected children, usually by the age of 16. Some children initially show a promising response to antiseizure medication (ASM), but around 80% develop medically intractable seizures.[11] Early referral to epilepsy surgical services is important (see Chapter 6).

Tuberous sclerosis is a genetic disorder that commonly causes malformations of cortical development. Cortical dysplasias, including tubers as well as subependymal nodules (see Figure 3.1d) and giant cell astrocytomas, provide an epileptogenic focus, with seizures occurring in most individuals before they are 1 year old.

Vascular malformations. Sturge–Weber syndrome is a vascular malformation with a genetic cause. It is characterized by a facial port-wine stain and an ipsilateral leptomeningeal angioma (vascular abnormality), which causes ischemia, atrophy, and calcification in the affected cortex. This causes seizures in 75–90% of patients, usually beginning in the first year of life.[12]

Other vascular problems that can result in epilepsy include arteriovenous malformation and cerebral angiomas.

Metabolic causes
Although most syndromes in CYPWE have a genetic basis, there are several metabolic conditions associated with the development of epilepsy that are conceptualized as a separate disorder.[13] These conditions usually start in early childhood. Recognition is important, as the most effective treatment usually involves correction of the underlying metabolic problem rather than ASM. Examples include pyridoxine-dependent epilepsy, glucose transporter (GLUT1)

deficiency, porphyria, aminoacidopathies, cerebral folate deficiency, and creatine disorders.

Immune-mediated causes
There is also a raft of antibody-mediated epilepsies, including anti-*N*-methyl-D-aspartate (NMDA) receptor encephalitis, α-amino-3-hydroxy-5-methyl-4-isoxazolepropionic acid (AMPA) receptor antibody, γ-aminobutyric acid B (GABA-B) antibody, and glutamic acid decarboxylase (GAD) 65 antibody. The clinical presentations vary, and much of the literature reports small case series. Focal-onset seizures developing to bilateral tonic-clonic seizures are the rule (70%).[14] Changes in mood, neurocognitive changes (particularly amnesia), and movement disorders are common comorbidities. Autoimmune encephalitis may be the presenting feature of a tumor that has triggered antibody production.

Antibody-mediated epilepsies are complex and varied. Detailed analysis is beyond the scope of this book, but diagnostic screening is discussed in Chapter 4. Treatment usually involves steroids and immunotherapy. Outcomes are variable. For example, children affected by voltage-gated potassium channel (VGKC) complex antibody encephalitis show a good response to immunotherapy, whereas those with GAD 65 autoimmune encephalitis generally have a poor outcome with both immunotherapy and ASM.

Infectious causes
Worldwide, infection is the commonest etiology for the development of epilepsy. Acute and/or chronic infection within the CNS can result in brain damage and seizures (most common in developing countries). Infectious causes include HIV, tuberculosis, malaria, bacterial meningitis, and viral meningitis. The more widespread the damage caused by these infections to the brain structure, the more difficult it is likely to be to control seizures. Treating the infection quickly is the most important therapeutic strategy.

Congenital cytomegalovirus (CMV) is asymptomatic in 85–90% of babies born with it,[15] but seizures, hydrocephalus, and cerebral palsy can occur in symptomatic cases, along with a myriad of other symptoms. Each child is unique, and it is difficult to predict the precise effects of CMV on an individual.

Neurocysticercosis is a parasitic infection caused by *Taenia solium*, a tapeworm found in pigs, and is one of the commonest symptomatic causes of epilepsy in sub-Saharan Africa, Latin America, and Asia.

Epilepsy with unknown etiology

Febrile infection-related epilepsy syndrome is a devastating condition with unknown pathogenesis despite extensive investigation. Seizures begin between the ages of 2 and 17 years (median 8 years) with rapid progression to refractory status epilepticus (SE). The mortality rate is high, and surviving patients require prolonged ventilator support and have cognitive and neurological impairment as well as ongoing seizures.

Rasmussen syndrome (RS) develops in previously normal children aged 1–10 years (peak 5–6 years). Intractable focal seizures, often including epilepsia partialis continua, develop along with a progressing hemiparesis and cognitive impairment. Neuroimaging reveals progressive hemispheric atrophy, the cause of which is unknown. Therefore, the pathology itself is the etiology of RS and so it is classified as an etiology-specific epilepsy syndrome.[16]

Triggers

Children or young people with established epilepsy have several environmental triggers for ongoing seizures (Table 3.2). The most

TABLE 3.2

Common seizure triggers in children and young people

- Sleep deprivation, particularly in children with sleep problems and autism
- Alcohol/illicit drugs (see Chapter 8)
- Prescribed medication that can alter the seizure threshold
- Intercurrent illness, particularly fever or diarrhea and vomiting
- Stress/anxiety
- Diet (irregular meals and excitotoxins)
- Specific triggers individual to the child
- Non-adherence to antiseizure medication

common is probably forgotten medication, particularly in teenagers who may also choose not to take medication because of peer pressure or perceived stigma. Viral or bacterial infections, particularly urinary tract infection, can trigger seizures due to pyrexia; the simple use of paracetamol (acetaminophen) can be very helpful. Heightened emotions, chiefly stress and anxiety but sometimes excitement, particularly in CYPWE with ID, can precipitate seizures. It is therefore very important not to ignore the child's psychosocial wellbeing when providing a holistic plan of care.

Disturbed sleep can also cause problems with seizure control, and there can be a complex interplay with some childhood epilepsies. For example, in developmental and/or epileptic encephalopathy with spike-and-wave activation in sleep (DEE-SWAS), epileptiform activity is significantly activated in sleep and may be associated with acquired cognitive and behavioral impairment.

Key points – causes and triggers

- There are numerous causes of pediatric epilepsy with etiologies broadly divided into structural, genetic, infectious, metabolic, immune, and unknown.
- A wide range of chromosomal and gene abnormalities are associated with childhood epilepsies.
- The most common structural causes of epilepsy are hippocampal sclerosis and traumatic or ischemic/hypoxic brain injury. High-quality cranial MRI is the investigation of choice for structural causes.
- Infection is the commonest cause of epilepsy. Treating the infection quickly is the most important therapeutic strategy.
- Non-adherence to ASM is the most common trigger for seizures in CYPWE.
- A thorough lifestyle assessment may identify triggers that can be addressed to dramatically reduce seizure burden and risk.

References

1. Altuna M, Gimenez S, Fortea J. Epilepsy in Down syndrome: a highly prevalent comorbidity. *J Clin Med* 2021;10:2776.
2. Rinaldi B, Vaisfeld A, Amarri S et al. Guideline recommendations for diagnosis and clinical management of Ring14 syndrome – first report of an ad hoc task force. *Orphanet J Rare Dis* 2017;12:69.
3. Whitney R, Nair A, McCready E et al. The spectrum of epilepsy in children with 15q13.3 microdeletion syndrome. *Seizure* 2021;92:221–9.
4. Hirsch E, French J, Scheffer IE et al. ILAE definition of the idiopathic generalized epilepsy syndromes: position paper by the ILAE Task Force on Nosology and Definitions. *Epilepsia* 2022;63:1475–99.
5. Blazekovic A, Jercic KG, Meglaj S et al. Genetics of pediatric epilepsy: next-generation sequencing in clinical practice. *Genes (Basel)* 2022;13:1466.
6. Barkovich MJ. Pediatric brain maturation and migration disorders. *Diagnostics* 2022;12:1123.
7. Wong-Kisiel LC, Britton JW, Witte RJ et al. Double inversion recovery magnetic resonance imaging in identifying focal cortical dysplasia. *Pediatr Neurol* 2016;61:87–93.
8. Radhakrishnan R, Verma S. Clinically relevant imaging in tuberous sclerosis. *J Clin Imaging Sci* 2011;1:39.
9. Nóbrega AW Jr, Gregory CP, Schlindwein-Zanini R et al. Mesial temporal lobe epilepsy with hippocampal sclerosis is infrequently associated with neuronal autoantibodies. *Epilepsia* 2018;59:e152–6.
10. Represa A. Why malformations of cortical development cause epilepsy. *Front Neurosci* 2019;13:250.
11. International League Against Epilepsy. *Structural Etiology: Malformations of Cortical Development.* epilepsydiagnosis.org/aetiology/malform-cortical-dev-overview.html, last accessed 1 November 2023.
12. Victorio MC. Neurocutaneous syndromes: Sturge-Weber syndrome. In: *MSD Manual Professional Version*, 2022 [online]. msdmanuals.com/en-gb/professional/pediatrics/neurocutaneous-syndromes/sturge-weber-syndrome, last accessed 1 November 2023.
13. Zuberi SM, Wirrell E, Yozawitz et al. ILAE classification and definition of epilepsy syndromes with onset in neonates and infants: position statement by the ILAE Task Force on Nosology and Definitions. *Epilepsia* 2022;63:1349–97.
14. Bakpa OD, Reuber M, Irani SR. Antibody-associated epilepsies: clinical features, evidence for immunotherapies and future research questions. *Seizure* 2016;41:26–41.

15. Akpan US, Pillarisetty LS. Congenital cytomegalovirus infection. *StatPearls [Internet].* StatPearls Publishing, 2023.

16. Riney K, Bogacz A, Somerville E et al. International League Against Epilepsy classification and definition of epilepsy syndromes with onset at a variable age: position paper by the ILAE Task Force on Nosology and Definitions. *Epilepsia* 2022;63:1443–74.

**Neurology and
Neuroscience**

4 Diagnosis

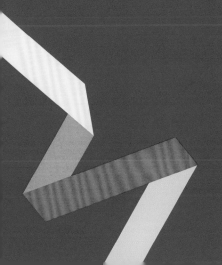

HEALTHCARE

When assessing a child or young person who presents with a seizure(s), three fundamental questions need to be addressed.
- Is/are the episode(s) epileptic seizure(s)?
- What is/are the seizure type(s)?
- Is there an identifiable epilepsy syndrome?

Particular seizure types respond better to particular antiseizure medications (ASM), and certain ASM are recommended for certain epilepsy syndromes, so if the evaluation does not progress further than the first question, the individual is likely to receive suboptimal treatment and management.

Children and young people are usually referred to an epilepsy clinic after attending the emergency department or via their primary care provider. In the UK, recommendations from the National Institute for Health and Care Excellence (NICE)[1] and the Scottish Intercollegiate Guidelines Network (SIGN)[2] state that the diagnosis of epilepsy should be made by an epilepsy specialist. In real terms, this is usually a pediatrician with a specialist interest in epilepsy. However, if there is any diagnostic doubt, referral to a tertiary pediatric neurologist may be required.

Diagnostic criteria
Epilepsy is defined as any of the following.
- At least two unprovoked (or reflex) seizures more than 24 hours apart.
- One unprovoked (or reflex) seizure and a probability of further seizures similar to the general recurrence risk (at least 60%) after two unprovoked seizures over the next 10 years.
- Diagnosis of an epilepsy syndrome.[3]

Despite advances in investigative techniques, the diagnosis of epilepsy remains a clinical one (Tables 4.1 and 4.2).[1,4–7]

Initial presentation
History. A detailed history is the single most important step in the diagnostic process. It is important to include any witnesses and, where developmentally appropriate, the child or young person.

TABLE 4.1

Initial tests and the information they can provide

- Initial presentation in an emergency department (or in clinic if not previously completed)
- Detailed history of initial event plus any subsequent events
- Medical history of child and family, plus details of any relevant impairment in learning or behavior
- ECG with calculation of QTc to rule out a potential cardiac cause for the paroxysmal event
- Blood pressure and blood glucose to rule out other causes
- Blood gas, calcium, and magnesium (in emergency department if not fully recovered)
- Baseline blood tests, plus specialist blood tests to rule out genetic, infectious, immune, or metabolic causes (in clinic or on ward, as indicated; see Table 4.2).

TABLE 4.2

Tests to identify specific etiologies

Etiology	Type of test	Reason for test
Infants (<2 years old)		
Neurophysio-logical	• EEG (routine and during sleep, interictal or ictal where possible)	To look for epileptiform activity or evidence of hypsarrhythmia or multifocal discharges, or background activity suggesting encephalopathy
Structural	• Brain MRI	To check for brain injury (e.g. HIE), abnormalities in brain development (e.g. focal cortical dysplasia), or demyelination
		May need to be repeated after the age of 2 years

CONTINUED

TABLE 4.2 CONTINUED

Tests to identify specific etiologies

Etiology	Type of test	Reason for test
Infants (<2 years old) *continued*		

Metabolic	• Bloods
	  – Biotinidase
	  – Plasma amino acids
	  – Plasma ammonia
	  – Lactate
	  – Calcium
	  – Magnesium
	  – Glucose
	  – Very-long-chain fatty acids for peroxisomal disorders
	• Urine
	  – Organic acids
	  – Urine purines and pyrimidines
	  – α-AASA
	  – Pipecolic acid
	  – Sulfite
	• Lumbar puncture
	  – CSF/serum glucose ratio
	  – CSF amino acids
	  – CSF neurotransmitters and pterins
	  – CSF lactate
		To check for potential metabolic causes or deficiencies, some of which may be treatable
		
		A basic metabolic screen should be completed, with further tests as guided by the pediatric neurology or metabolic teams
		
		For further information on individual tests see *Vademecum Metabolicum* at vademetab.org

Genetic	• Bloods
	  – CGH
	  – Karyotyping
	  – Exome sequencing
	  – Whole genome sequencing
		To check for genetic causes or metabolic conditions causing epilepsy

CONTINUED

TABLE 4.2 CONTINUED

Etiology	Type of test	Reason for test
Infectious	• Routine blood tests • Lumbar puncture with usual caution – CSF, including lactate and oligoclonal bands	To check for encephalitis or meningitis Paired serum and CSF testing is useful for any inflammation including autoimmune encephalitis
Children and young people		
Neurophysiological	• EEG (routine/sleep deprived ± melatonin)	To look for generalized epileptiform discharges or identify a likely area of focal discharges
Cardiac	• 12-lead ECG, with evaluation of QTc	To rule out possible cardiac causes for paroxysmal episodes or for those with known channelopathies Refer to cardiologist if any history of cardiac issues
Structural	• Brain MRI	For focal seizures and all seizures that fail to respond to treatment For CYPWE who do not have expected clinical progress, to identify any structural changes/abnormalities Not usually required in recognized focal childhood syndromes
Metabolic	• Bloods • Urine • Lumbar puncture (see Infants above)	Consider in children with multidrug-resistant epilepsy, developmental delay, regression, or multiseizure types who have not previously had metabolic tests

CONTINUED

TABLE 4.2 CONTINUED

Tests to identify specific etiologies

Etiology	Type of test	Reason for test
Children and young people *continued*		
Genetic	• Bloods – CGH – Whole genome sequencing	To check for genetic causes in children with multidrug-resistant epilepsy, developmental delay, regression, or multiseizure types who have not previously had genetic tests
Immune	• Bloods – Autoimmune encephalitis screen for antibodies to NMDA, CASPR2, LGI1, VGKC, MOG, GABA, and AMPA receptors • Also consider SLE as a cause: – ESR – ANA – anti-dsDNA	For onset of a new neuropsychiatric disorder and/or sudden progressive seizures To identify immune-related encephalopathies
Infectious	• Bloods • Lumbar puncture with usual caution (see Infants above)	To identify encephalitis or meningitis

α-AASA, α-aminoadipic semialdehyde; AMPA, α-amino-3-hydroxy-5-methyl-4-isoxazolepropionic acid; ANA, antinuclear antibodies; CASPR2, contactin-associated protein-like 2; CGH, comparative genomic hybridization, also known as chromosomal microarray analysis (CMA); CSF, cerebrospinal fluid; CYPWE, children and young people with epilepsy; dsDNA, double-stranded DNA; ECG, electrocardiogram; EEG, electroencephalogram; ESR, erythrocyte sedimentation rate; GABA, γ-aminobutyric acid; HIE, hypoxic ischemic encephalopathy; LGI1, leucine-rich glioma-inactivated 1; MOG, myelin oligodendrocyte glycoprotein; MRI, magnetic resonance imaging; NMDA, N-methyl-D-aspartate; SLE, systemic lupus erythematosus; VGKC, voltage-gated potassium channel complex.

Compiled from information in National Institute for Health and Care Excellence (NICE) guidelines and International League Against Epilepsy (ILAE) position papers on the classification and definition of epilepsy syndromes.[1,4–7]

History taking in epilepsy should focus as much on what occurs before and after a seizure as the actual seizure itself. Many paroxysmal episodes can mimic an epileptic seizure. Table 4.3 provides strategies for history taking. Note the emphasis on context, as well as symptoms before and after the seizure.

TABLE 4.3

History taking from events before, during, and after a seizure

A	Antecedent	• Events in the previous 24 hours
		• Any triggers/warning/aura (e.g. feeling unwell, a late night, missed doses of ASM)
C	Context	• Where did it happen?
		• What was the child doing?
		• What time of day did it occur?
		• If nocturnal, was the child awake, going to sleep, or waking up, or did it occur during sleep?
O	Onset	• What was the first thing observed when the seizure started?
		• Was there any change in skin color?
P	Progression	• What happened next?
		• Did the child fall to the ground? If so, how?
		• Was the child responsive?
		• What happened to the child's eyes?
		• Were there any movements of the child's face/body (e.g. shaking, jerking, eyelid flickering)? If yes, state what/where
		• Did it start on one side or symmetrically?
		• Was there a change in the child's breathing pattern?
		• If there were multiple phases, how long did each one last?

CONTINUED

TABLE 4.3 CONTINUED

History taking from events before, during, and after a seizure

E	End	• Was the child stiff or floppy?
		• When did the event end? Try to distinguish between the end of the seizure and any postictal phase
		• How long did the seizure last (estimated or timed)?
		• Was there any change in skin color?
		• Was the child incontinent?
		• Did the child vomit?
A	After	• How was the child after the seizure?
		• In the postictal phase, was the child tired or confused, or did they need to sleep?
		• How long did it take the child to return to normal?
		• Was the child given any medication to stop the seizure?
		• What did the parent/witness do during and after the seizure?

ASM, antiseizure medication.
Adapted from Luton & Dunstable University Hospital's Seizure Integrated Care Pathway Paediatric Assessment Unit Admission Form, which uses the mnemonic ACOPEA.[8]

If there is more than one type of seizure, each seizure should be described separately.

Seizure diaries. Asking families or young people to keep a seizure diary of any paroxysmal events is essential. This should include anything that may have precipitated the event, how the event started and progressed, how the event ended, and the period after the event. Seizure diaries may also help to identify any patterns in the events, as well as providing a record of any clear improvement or deterioration of the events in relation to any treatments/medications.

Forms such as the CEWT (Children's Epilepsy Workstream in Trent [UK]) seizure description sheet (Table 4.4) can provide questions that will aid/prompt witnesses to recall this information or know what to look out for before, during, and after any future events.[9]

TABLE 4.4

Questions to aid accurate seizure recording

Question
Who witnessed the episode?
Date and time of episode?
Did you notice anything before the episode?
What was the child doing just before the episode started? Did anything appear to trigger it?
How did the episode start?
Was there any change in the child's breathing or color?
What happened next? (There are many possibilities. Try to note down as much as you can.) • Did the child lose consciousness? • Was the child able to respond to you? • Was the child's body floppy or stiff? • Did the child's arms and legs move? • What did the movements look like? • Were the child's eyes open or closed? • Did the child's head or eyes jerk or go to one side? Which side?
How long did the episode last and how did you know it had finished?
What was the child like after the episode (e.g. drowsy, sleepy, aggressive)?
How long was it until the child was back to their usual self?
Any other comments?

Adapted from the Children's Epilepsy Workstream in Trent (CEWT) Epilepsy-To-Go Seizure Description sheet.[9]

Video diaries. The availability of phones with video capabilities has proved invaluable in providing clear unbiased visual recording of events. Videos of paroxysmal events significantly improve the chance of a correct diagnosis of epilepsy and seizure semiology. They are also helpful in differentiating other non-epileptic events. Issues such as receiving, storage, and consent should be considered, especially where videos may be shared with specialist services for diagnostic support.[10] Companies such as V-Create and Isla have developed software to meet some of these challenges.

Electroencephalography is a useful diagnostic tool in epilepsy, but a normal or abnormal EEG alone cannot be used to rule out or diagnose epilepsy. This is especially true in children as their brains are still developing: 2–4% of otherwise healthy children and young people will have an abnormal EEG with no correlating clinical symptoms. This number can rise to 10–30% when a cerebral pathology is present.[11] Conversely, up to 50% of EEGs will be normal or show non-specific abnormalities (generally defined as non-contributary) in children who have had an epileptic seizure. However, an EEG can be useful in determining seizure type or identifying an epilepsy syndrome.

Routine EEGs are often non-contributary as they offer only a short period of recording, usually during an interictal period. Activation techniques, including hyperventilation and photic stimulation (Figure 4.1), can be helpful in uncovering abnormalities. Hyperventilation can be difficult to obtain in younger children or those with significant intellectual disability (ID). Diagnostic yield may also be increased by repeat recordings. If the initial EEG is unremarkable and the diagnosis remains in doubt, a sleep-deprivation study is recommended.

Routine EEGs have a limited role in determining whether ASM can be safely tapered after a prolonged seizure-free interval; response to treatment and syndromic classification are more reliable indicators.[12]

Sleep-deprivation study. If the initial EEG is unremarkable and the diagnosis remains in doubt, a sleep-deprivation study is recommended, particularly in the case of suspected genetic generalized epilepsy (GGE)

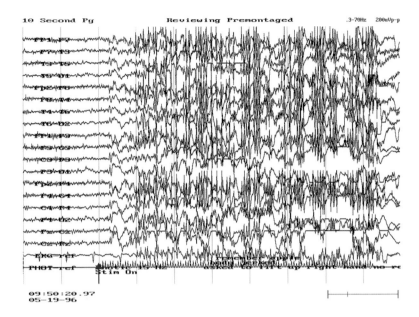

Figure 4.1 Photoconvulsive response provoked by intermittent photic stimulation. The arrow shows when photic stimulation began.

where it is mandated if the routine recording is non-contributary. It may be difficult to get children to sleep or settle in an unfamiliar setting. If that is the case, the use of melatonin may increase the likelihood of obtaining EEG recordings during sleep.[13]

Ambulatory (portable) EEG is also available to allow prolonged recording in the home environment. On the plus side, this allows recording to take place in the child's usual environment, but technical faults are more likely and accurate correlation with simultaneous behaviors on video is available only with certain recording systems. It also relies on the patient or caregiver activating the camera, something that many, surprisingly, fail to do.

Video telemetry is the gold standard in EEG recording but is not widely available in local hospitals and may require referral to a specialist/tertiary service center. It is especially useful where there is diagnostic doubt. Video footage of reported events can be reviewed to check if there are correlating epileptiform discharges.

Genetic testing

Our understanding of the underlying genetic causes for certain epilepsy syndromes has increased exponentially over the last couple of decades. Many of the conditions mentioned in Chapter 2 have a genetic basis. Comparative genomic hybridization (CGH) arrays, epilepsy gene panels, and whole genome sequencing are becoming more readily available in many countries.

However, before embarking on genetic testing, children and young people with epilepsy (CYPWE) and their families or caregivers should be counseled about the purpose of the test and the possible implication of the results. Whole genome assays may identify abnormalities other than epilepsy, which may in turn require testing of other family members.[1] Furthermore, many countries conduct active genetic research. It is important for clinicians to understand the local consent process for this, including storage of samples (blood, saliva, tissue, etc.), processes for the analysis and use of samples, and mechanisms for withdrawing consent in the future.

Not all CYPWE will require genetic assays. UK guidelines provide a succinct list of indications for testing (Table 4.5).[1] Individuals with other conditions that may cause seizures should also be tested, and full lists of these are available in a number of international databases.[14,15]

TABLE 4.5

Indications for genetic testing

- Under 2 years old when seizures started
- Clinical features suggestive of a specific epilepsy syndrome
- Additional clinical features
  - intellectual disability
  - autism spectrum disorder
  - structural abnormalities, such as dysmorphia or congenital malformations
  - unexplained cognitive or memory decline

Accurate diagnosis of genetic epilepsies allows for the optimization of treatment modalities. For example, the use of cannabidiol or the ketogenic diet in children with Dravet syndrome, or large doses of pyridoxine (vitamin B6) in pyridoxine-dependent epilepsy, a condition that is always resistant to ASM.[16]

Imaging

Magnetic resonance imaging (MRI) is the most sensitive imaging modality for detecting structural abnormalities in the brain that may be causing seizures in some children.[1]

The criteria for MRI in CYPWE are:
- newly diagnosed epilepsy in a child under 2 years old
- epilepsy with focal onset (unless there is evidence of childhood epilepsy with centrotemporal spikes)
- failure of first-line ASM.

However, access to MRI facilities and appropriate pediatric reporting are variable. Issues such as the ability of a child or young person to keep still for a prolonged period of time, the need for/ availability of sedation, or facilities for general anesthetic also need to be considered.

Computed tomography (CT) should be considered if MRI is not available or is unsuitable because of the need for sedation or general anesthetic. CT should be used in acute situations if seizures could be caused by an acute illness or neurological lesion.

Further imaging. For CYPWE who are eligible for epilepsy surgery, functional MRI (fMRI), positron emission tomography (PET), single photon emission computed tomography (SPECT), or magnetoencephalography (MEG) may provide further information. These are generally only available at specialist centers.

Differential diagnoses

The International League Against Epilepsy (ILAE) has split the imitators of epilepsy into six categories.

- Syncope and anoxic seizures, including vasovagal syncope, reflex anoxic seizures, breath-holding attacks, hyperventilation syncope, and long QT and cardiac syncope.
- Behavioral, psychological, and psychiatric disorders, including daydreaming/inattention, self-gratification, panic attacks, dissociative states, functional seizures (see Chapter 10), hallucinations in psychiatric disorders, and fabricated/fictitious illness.
- Sleep-related conditions, including sleep-related rhythmic movement disorders, hypnogogic jerks, parasomnias, rapid eye movement (REM) sleep disorders, benign neonatal sleep myoclonus, and narcolepsy-cataplexy.
- Paroxysmal movement disorders, including tics, stereotypies, paroxysmal kinesigenic dyskinesia, and episodic ataxias.
- Migraine-associated disorders, including migraine with visual aura, familial hemiplegic migraine, and cyclic vomiting.
- Miscellaneous events, including benign myoclonus of infancy and shuddering attacks, jitteriness, Sandifer syndrome, and raised intracranial pressure.

Globally, misdiagnosis rates of epilepsy are high, so it is important that these disorders are considered when evaluating paroxysmal events. It should also be noted that epileptic and non-epileptic disorders can coexist in some individuals. Further information, including important discriminating features for these disorders, can be found at epilepsydiagnosis.org/epilepsy-imitators.html.[3]

'Do we have a definite diagnosis, and can we put a name to it?'

The aim is to answer the questions that were posed at the beginning of this chapter (see page 52). If a diagnosis of epilepsy can be confirmed and the seizure types (see Chapter 1), or epilepsy syndrome (see Chapter 2) identified, then CYPWE and their caregivers can be given more helpful information. This can include likely prognosis and preferred treatment or management options, including which ASM are more suitable for the diagnosed seizure type(s) or syndrome and which medications should be avoided.

Important questions, such as the likelihood of seizure freedom and whether treatment is expected to be needed in childhood only or is likely to continue into adolescence or adulthood, can also be addressed.

The British Paediatric Neurology Association (BPNA) has suggested the DESSCRIBE mnemonic as a useful tool. It encompasses an initial description of events and whether they indicate epilepsy, and considers seizure type, possible syndrome, and any identifiable or presumed cause. It also encourages those working with CYPWE to holistically consider associated behavioral, emotional, or educational impairments (Figure 4.2).[17]

Criteria for referral to a tertiary service

Tertiary services in pediatric epilepsy can be defined as being led by a 'pediatric neurologist who devotes the majority of their working time to epilepsy, is working in a multidisciplinary tertiary referral center with appropriate diagnostic and therapeutic resources, and is subject to regular peer review'.

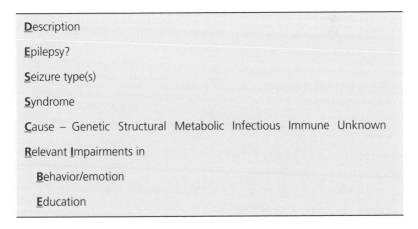

Figure 4.2 British Paediatric Neurology Association (BPNA) Paediatric Epilepsy Training DESSCRIBE tool is a useful means of obtaining a description of events and any identifiable or presumed cause.

International guidelines on the management of CYPWE recommend that referral to tertiary services should be considered when one or more of the following criteria are present.[1,18]

- The epilepsy is not controlled with medication within 2 years of onset.
- Management is unsuccessful after two drugs.
- The child is under 2 years old.
- The child or young person experiences, or is at risk of, unacceptable side effects from medication.
- There is a unilateral structural lesion.
- There is psychological or psychiatric comorbidity.
- There is diagnostic doubt as to the nature of the seizures or the seizure syndrome.

Supporting families and parents

Explaining epilepsy. It is important that families receive both verbal and written information regarding their epilepsy diagnosis and prognosis. Verbal and written information should also be given regarding any suggested treatment options. If seizure first aid and seizure safety, including information about heights, water, and road safety, have not previously been discussed, these should also be included. Sudden unexpected death in epilepsy (SUDEP) should also be discussed at an early stage. Contact details for the epilepsy team/ epilepsy nurses should be provided for any queries or concerns after the initial diagnosis.

Getting the right support. Families can find it helpful to be in contact with others who are going through, or have previously navigated, an epilepsy diagnosis. Information about local or national support groups, such as Epilepsy Action (UK, Australia), Young Epilepsy (UK), or Epilepsy Foundation (USA, Australia), can be provided.

Witnessing epileptic seizures and dealing with a diagnosis of epilepsy can have a significant effect on the whole family. Access to a clinical psychologist, where available, can help families come to terms with this change in family life.

Key points – diagnosis

- Diagnosis should be made by a pediatric neurologist or a pediatrician with a specialist interest in epilepsy.
- There is no definitive diagnostic test for epilepsy. A detailed clinical history with video recordings offers the best prospect for accurate diagnosis.
- An EEG, imaging, and blood tests may help to identify the type of seizure, epilepsy syndrome, or underlying cause of the seizures.
- Referral to tertiary services is required for children under 2 years old, any child or young person where diagnostic doubt exists, individuals who are eligible for epilepsy surgery, CYPWE whose seizures are not controlled by two or more ASM, and CYPWE with psychological or psychiatric comorbidities.
- Both verbal and written information should be provided for families dealing with a diagnosis of epilepsy.
- Epilepsy nurses and local and national epilepsy groups can provide vital support for families.
- Therapy or clinical psychology should be considered to support the whole family after a diagnosis of epilepsy.

References

1. National Institute for Health and Care Excellence (NICE). *Epilepsies in children, young people and adults. NICE guideline [NG217]*. NICE, 2022. nice.org. uk/guidance/ng217

2. Scottish Intercollegiate Guidelines Network (SIGN). *SIGN 159. Epilepsies in children and young people: investigative procedures and management. A national clinical guideline*. SIGN, 2021. sign.ac.uk/ media/1844/sign-159-epilepsy- in-children-final.pdf

3. International League Against Epilepsy (ILAE). *EpilepsyDiagnosis.org. Diagnostic Manual*. ILAE, 2022. epilepsydiagnosis.org, last accessed 1 November 2023.

4. Zuberi SM, Wirrell E, Yozawitz E et al. ILAE classification and definition of epilepsy syndromes with onset in neonates and infants: position statement by the ILAE Task Force on Nosology and Definitions. *Epilepsia* 2022;63:1349–97.

5. Specchio N, Wirrell EC, Scheffer IE et al. International League Against Epilepsy classification and definition of epilepsy syndromes with onset in childhood: position paper by the ILAE Task Force on Nosology and Definitions. *Epilepsia* 2022;63:1398–442.

6. Riney K, Bogacz A, Somerville E et al. International League Against Epilepsy classification and definition of epilepsy syndromes with onset at a variable age: position statement by the ILAE Task Force on Nosology and Definitions. *Epilepsia* 2022;63:1443–74.

7. Hirsch E, French J, Scheffer IE et al. ILAE definition of the idiopathic generalized epilepsy syndromes: position statement by the ILAE Task Force on Nosology and Definitions. *Epilepsia* 2022;63:1475–99.

8. Luton & Dunstable University Hospital. *Seizure Integrated Care Pathway Paediatric Assessment Unit Admission Form*. eqip.rcpch. ac.uk/wp-content/uploads/ sites/19/2021/05/luton_seizure_ admission_document_apr.pdf, last accessed 1 November 2023.

9. Children's Epilepsy Workstream in Trent (CEWT). *Comprehensive Care Plan Resources: Seizure Description*. CEWT, 2008. cewt.org.uk/CEWT/ Epilepsy-to-go.html

10. Ricci L, Boscarino M, Assenza G et al. Epilepsy Study Group of the Italian Neurological Society. Clinical utility of home videos for diagnosing epileptic seizures: a systematic review and practical recommendations for optimal and safe recording. *Neurol Sci* 2021;42:1301–9.

11. Smith SJM. EEG in the diagnosis, classification, and management of patients with epilepsy. *J Neurol Neurosurg Psychiatr* 2005;76(Suppl II):ii2–ii7.

12. Bessant P, Chadwick D, Eaton B et al. Randomised study of antiepileptic drug withdrawal in patients in remission. Medical Research Council Antiepileptic Drug Withdrawal Study Group. *Lancet* 1991;337:1175–80.

13. Alix JJP, Kandler RH, Pang C et al. Sleep deprivation and melatonin for inducing sleep in paediatric electroencephalography: a prospective multicentre service evaluation. *Dev Med Child Neurol* 2019;61:181–5.

14. NHS England. *National Genomic Test Directory*. NHS England, 2018 (updated 2023). england. nhs.uk/publication/national-genomic-test-directories, last accessed 1 November 2023.

15. National Institutes of Health (NIH) National Library of Medicine. *National Genomic Test Directory. GTR: Genetic Testing Registry*. NIH, 2023. ncbi.nlm.nih.gov/gtr, last accessed 1 November 2023.

16. Coughlin CR 2nd, Tseng LA, Abdenur JE et al. Consensus guidelines for the diagnosis and management of pyridoxine-dependent epilepsy due to α-aminoadipic semialdehyde dehydrogenase deficiency. *J Inherit Metab Dis* 2021; 44:178–92.

17. British Paediatric Neurology Association (BPNA). *Paediatric Epilepsy Training (PET)*. courses.bpna.org.uk/index.php?page=paediatric-epilepsy-training, last accessed 1 November 2023.

18. Kwan P, Arzimanoglou A, Berg AT et al. Definition of drug resistant epilepsy: consensus proposal by the ad hoc Task Force of the ILAE Commission on Therapeutic Strategies. *Epilepsia* 2010;51:1069–77.

5 Pharmacological treatment

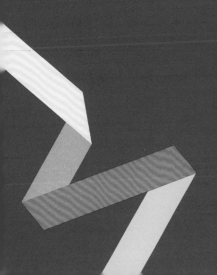

HEALTHCARE

Management principles

How does antiseizure medication work? Antiseizure medications (ASM) work in different ways to prevent seizures, either by decreasing excitation or enhancing inhibition of neurons. Sometimes the mode of action is unknown when the ASM is launched, or it changes when the drug is analyzed in more detail in postmarketing studies.[1] Important modes of action include:

- altering chemical activity in the neurons by affecting sodium, calcium, or potassium ion channels in the cell membrane
- altering chemical transmission between neurons by affecting γ-aminobutyric acid (GABA) or glutamate neurotransmitters in the synapses.

When should antiseizure medication be used? ASM should be prescribed for children and young people with epilepsy (CYPWE) when they have experienced two or more seizures. Some provoked seizures (such as those associated with photosensitivity or concomitant illness), self-limited epilepsy with centrotemporal spikes (SeLECTS), and seizures associated with metabolic disturbances may be managed with avoidant activity or by treating the underlying metabolic disorder. These approaches do not always require ASM.

The decision to start ASM (or not) should be made after a full discussion with the child or young person and their parents/caregivers, including the risks and benefits of treatment. Information should be presented about the risk of seizure recurrence, the chance of remission of seizures, and the likely duration of treatment, which can range from a few years for childhood absence epilepsy (CAE) to lifelong for juvenile myoclonic epilepsy (JME).

Explaining the risks and benefits. At the onset of treatment, common and uncommon but serious side effects, such as hypersensitivity reactions, should be carefully explained. For CYPWE who are likely to need ASM during at least some of their reproductive life, the potential teratogenicity and effects on fertility and interactions with hormonal contraceptives need to be discussed. Although the focus of these discussions has concentrated on information for young women, ASM can cause impotence in men and affect sperm count and motility. Evidence is emerging of a risk for some malformations in children whose fathers took ASM, particularly sodium valproate, and even an intergenerational risk requires careful discussion despite the urgent need for further research in this area.[2]

The importance of adherence to prescribed medication to minimize the chance of breakthrough seizures, thereby reducing the risk of injury and even sudden unexpected death (SUDEP) due to poor seizure control, should be discussed and revisited, particularly with CYPWE whose seizure control is suboptimal. Written information about ASM, including 'easy read' literature where available, should be provided when ASM is initiated.[3]

Treatment selection. Deciding on the most appropriate treatment for seizures will depend on the individual's age, sex, and weight, taking into consideration the type of seizures (Table 5.1), concomitant medication, and underlying health conditions. Consideration should also be given to the potential longevity of the epilepsy diagnosis when choosing an ASM.[3]

Monitoring effectiveness. ASM effectiveness is assessed by monitoring efficacy and tolerability. ASM should be started at low doses and titrated slowly, usually on a weekly or 2-weekly basis depending on which ASM is chosen, to establish an effective regimen. Slow titration helps to avoid concentration-dependent side effects, prevents sedation or cognitive impairments, and ensures early detection of hypersensitivity rashes and hepatotoxicity.[3]

Managing treatment effects. Measuring serum ASM concentrations can provide information on the child or young person's adherence to treatment and helps to minimize the potential for side effects and neurotoxicity, which can occur below, within, or above therapeutic ranges. However, routine measurement of ASM concentration is not indicated for most CYPWE. If seizures continue, then treatment should be increased within the limits of tolerability with the aim of achieving complete seizure freedom.[3]

Changing treatments. Alternative treatments should be discussed and initiated if seizure control remains poor. To prevent breakthrough seizures, second-line treatments should be titrated

TABLE 5.1

Efficacy of selected antiseizure medication against common seizure types and syndromes

ASM	Type of seizure/syndrome					
	Focal	Focal to bilateral tonic–clonic	Tonic–clonic	Absence	Myoclonic	Lennox–Gastaut
CBZ	+	+	+	−	−	?
CEN	+	+	+	?	?	?
ESM	−	−	−	+	−	−
LCM	+	+	+	?	?	?
LEV	+	+	+	?+	+	?
LTG	+	+	+	+	+*	+
OXC	+	+	+	−	−	0
PER	+	+	?	?	?	?
RFN	+	+	+	+	?	+
TGB	+	+	?	−	?	?
TPM	+	+	+	?	+	+
VGB	+	+	?	−	−	?
VPA	+	+	+	+	+	+
ZNS	+	+	+	?+	+	?+

*Lamotrigine may worsen myoclonic seizures in some cases. + proven efficacy; ?+ probable efficacy; 0 ineffective; − worsens control; ? unknown. ASM, antiseizure medication; CBZ, carbamazepine; CEN, cenobamate; ESM, ethosuximide; LCM, lacosamide; LEV, levetiracetam; LTG, lamotrigine; OXC, oxcarbazepine; PER, perampanel; RFN, rufinamide; TGB, tiagabine; TPM, topiramate; VGB, vigabatrin; VPA, sodium valproate; ZNS, zonisamide.

into the current drug regimen before considering withdrawal of the failed medication. Where possible, monotherapy should be used to try to prevent drug-to-drug interactions, although some CYPWE will need polytherapy.[3]

Withdrawing treatments. ASM should be withdrawn if it is clearly ineffective or if the child or young person is experiencing significant side effects that are detrimental to their health. For example, Stevens–Johnson syndrome is a potentially life-threatening side effect, characterized by a rash in its early stages. It is particularly associated with lamotrigine and carbamazepine, although it can occur with all ASM. This is especially important when treating CYPWE of Han Chinese, Japanese, or European origin. Some ASM may cause deterioration in mood or behavior in CYPWE where there was no previous concern (Table 5.2); choosing an alternative ASM would be advantageous for these individuals.

It may also be appropriate to withdraw ASM after a suitable period of seizure freedom. In CYPWE, this is often considered to be 2 years, although evidence suggests that 5 years is optimal in adults.[3] It should also be remembered that some epilepsies will remit after a certain age, while others are lifelong.

TABLE 5.2

Adverse effects of ASM on cognition and behavior

ASM	Cognitive	Behavioral
BRV	0	0
CBZ	+	0
CEN	^	^
CLB	+	+
CZP	++	+
ESL	0	0
ESM	+	+
FBM	0	+

CONTINUED

TABLE 5.2 CONTINUED

Adverse effects of ASM on cognition and behavior

ASM	Cognitive	Behavioral
FEN	?	+
GBP	0	0
LCM	0	0
LEV	0	+
LTG	0	0
OXC	+?	0
PB	++	++
PER	0	+?*
PGB	0	0
PHT	+	0
PRM	++	++
RFN	0	0
TGB	0	0
TPM	+*	+
VGB	0	+
VPA	+	0
ZNS	0	+

*Risk reduced by slow titration. ^ limited real world data; 0 no effect; ? unknown; +? possible effect; + mild effect; ++ marked effect.

BRV, brivaracetam; CBZ, carbamazepine; CEN, cenobamate; CLB, clobazam; CZP, clonazepam; ESL, eslicarbazepine acetate; ESM, ethosuximide; FBM, felbamate; FEN, fenfluramine; GBP, gabapentin; LCM, lacosamide; LEV, levetiracetam; LTG, lamotrigine; OXC, oxcarbazepine; PB, phenobarbital; PER, perampanel; PGB, pregabalin; PHT, phenytoin; PRM, primidone; RFN, rufinamide; TGB, tiagabine; TPM, topiramate; VGB, vigabatrin; VPA, sodium valproate; ZNS, zonisamide.

Antiseizure medications

As discussed above, selection of ASM in CYPWE depends on the type of seizures and/or epilepsy syndrome, age, sex, and weight, as well as any concomitant medication and underlying health conditions. The key features of ASM used to treat CYPWE are summarized below.[4]

For full prescribing information, please consult the product labeling approved in your country.

Brivaracetam

Indications. Adjunctive treatment for focal-onset seizures with or without bilateral tonic-clonic seizures.

Mechanism of action. Binds to SV2A. The exact role of this protein has yet to be elucidated, but it has been shown to modulate the exocytosis of neurotransmitters.

Dose and administration. By mouth, intravenous injection, or intravenous infusion. Tablets (10 mg, 25 mg, 50 mg, 75 mg, 100 mg), oral solution (10 mg/mL), intravenous injection (50 mg/5 mL).

- 2–17 years (bodyweight 10–19 kg): starting dose 0.5–1.25 mg/kg bd adjusted according to response; maintenance dose 1.25 mg/kg bd (maximum per dose 2.5 mg/kg bd).
- 2–17 years (bodyweight 20–49 kg): starting dose 0.5–1 mg/kg bd adjusted according to response; maintenance dose 1 mg/kg bd (maximum per dose 2 mg/kg bd).
- 2–17 years (bodyweight ≥50 kg): starting dose 25–50 mg bd adjusted according to response; maintenance dose 50 mg bd (maximum per dose 100 mg bd).

Contraindications. Rare hereditary galactose intolerance, total lactase deficiency, or glucose-galactose malabsorption.

Most common side effects. Anxiety, decreased appetite, constipation, cough, depression, dizziness, drowsiness, fatigue, increased risk of infection, insomnia, irritability, nausea, vertigo, and vomiting.

Significant interactions with carbamazepine and phenytoin.

Tips to aid adherence. As with most ASM, slow titration rates reduce the potential for side effects. Brivaracetam can be rapidly titrated in urgent clinical situations, but a more conservative approach is warranted in most CYPWE. Brivaracetam is better tolerated than levetiracetam (the only other ASM with a similar mode of action) in terms of psychiatric effects.

Other considerations. Brivaracetam is often used to replace levetiracetam when the latter shows promising seizure control but is not well tolerated, particularly if the child or young person experiences psychiatric side effects. The swap can be made without weaning levetiracetam and introducing brivaracetam, but the ratio needs to be considered (10:1 or 15:1) as it is not dose equivalent.

Cannabidiol

Indications. Adjunctive treatment for Lennox–Gastaut syndrome (LGS) or Dravet syndrome (DS). Some territories, including the UK and Europe, mandate concomitant use of Clobazam in the indication. Adjunctive therapy for seizures associated with tuberous sclerosis complex (TSC).

Mechanism of action. The precise mechanism of action is unknown. Cannabidiol does not interact with cannabinoid receptors. It reduces neuronal hyperexcitability through modulation of intracellular calcium via G protein-coupled receptor 55 and transient receptor potential vanilloid 1 channels. It also modulates adenosine-mediated signaling through inhibition of adenosine cellular uptake via the equilibrative nucleoside transporter 1.

Dose and administration. By mouth. Oral solution (100 mg/mL).

- 2–17 years: starting dose 2.5 mg/kg bd for 1 week, then increased to 5 mg/kg bd, with further increments of 2.5 mg/kg bd not faster than weekly, adjusted according to response; maximum dose 20 mg/kg/day (LGS and DS) or 25 mg/kg/day (TSC).

Contraindications. Hepatocellular injury. Avoid in patients with transaminase elevations greater than three times the upper limit of normal (ULN) and bilirubin greater than two times the ULN.

Most common side effects. Diarrhea and vomiting. Dosing around food is important (see below). Other side effects include hypersensitivity rashes (may require rapid drug discontinuation if serious), reduced appetite with weight reduction, neurotoxic effects such as tiredness, increased liver enzymes, irritability, and urinary tract infections.

Significant interactions. Carbamazepine may reduce plasma concentrations of cannabidiol by 30–60%. Clobazam substantially increases the active substances of cannabidiol, enhancing the therapeutic effects but also increasing the risk of neurotoxicity, necessitating clobazam dose adjustment. Sodium valproate significantly increases the risk of elevated transaminase levels, diarrhea, and decreased appetite; dose adjustment of sodium valproate, and in some cases discontinuation, may be required.

Theoretical risks of interaction with stiripentol, lamotrigine, and phenytoin: monitor carefully. Rifampicin, enzalutamide, mitotane, and

St John's wort may reduce cannabidiol levels significantly: dose adjustment may be required. Drugs affecting the substrates CYP1A2, CYP2B6, CYP2C8, CYP2C9, CYP2C19, UGT1A9, and UGT2B7 (for example, morphine, lorazepam, warfarin, and caffeine) may cause clinically significant interactions, though few have been studied: monitor carefully.

Tips to aid adherence. Cannabidiol should be administered with food, preferably similar types of food each time (for example, if taken with cereal at breakfast, the patient should take it with cereal each time, not a cooked breakfast or toast). This will increase its bioavailability (and therefore its therapeutic effect) and reduce the incidence of diarrhea, which can be severe. Gastrointestinal disturbances are more common with concomitant administration of sodium valproate. Many patients will be on dual therapy with sodium valproate: careful dose adjustments may be necessary to obtain optimal effects with minimal adverse reactions.

Carbamazepine

Indications. Focal-onset seizures and focal to bilateral tonic-clonic seizures and generalized tonic-clonic seizures (GTCS).

Mechanism of action. Enhancement of sodium channel inactivation by reducing high-frequency repetitive firing of action potentials.

Dose and administration. By mouth or rectum. Sustained- and immediate-release tablets (100 mg, 200 mg, 400 mg), oral suspension (100 mg/5 mL), suppositories (125 mg, 250 mg; short-term use only).
- By mouth
  - 1 month to 11 years: starting dose 5 mg/kg at night or 2.5 mg/kg bd, increasing by 2.5–5 mg/kg every 3–7 days as required; maintenance dose 5 mg/kg bd or tid; maximum dose 20 mg/kg/day.
  - 12–17 years: starting dose 100–200 mg od or bd, increasing slowly to 200–400 mg bd or tid depending on response; maximum dose 1.8 g/day.
- By rectum. Up to 250 mg up to four times a day for short-term use (maximum 7 days) when oral therapy is temporarily not possible; use approximately 25% more than the oral dose.

Contraindications. Acute porphyrias, atrioventricular (AV) conduction abnormalities (unless paced), and a history of bone marrow suppression.

Most common side effects. Allergic skin reactions, aplastic anemia, ataxia, blood disorders, blurring of vision, dermatitis, dizziness, drowsiness, dry mouth, edema, eosinophilia, fatigue, headache, hemolytic anemia, hyponatremia, leucopenia, nausea, unsteadiness, urticaria, and vomiting.

Significant interactions. Fosphenytoin, oxcarbazepine, phenobarbital, phenytoin, primidone, possibly clonazepam, and herbal remedies such as St John's wort reduce carbamazepine plasma levels, potentially requiring dose adjustments. Vigabatrin increases carbamazepine plasma concentrations. Primidone and sodium valproate increase plasma levels of the carbamazepine metabolite carbamazepine epoxide; this should be considered if clinical neurotoxicity occurs.

Carbamazepine induces metabolism of clobazam, clonazepam, ethosuximide, lamotrigine, eslicarbazepine acetate, oxcarbazepine, primidone, tiagabine, topiramate, sodium valproate, and zonisamide, potentially requiring an increase in dose.

Pharmacodynamic interactions can also be important with carbamazepine, particularly with levetiracetam where symptoms of carbamazepine toxicity may present. The oral contraceptive pill (OCP) is likely to be ineffective when used concomitantly with carbamazepine. The progesterone contraceptive implant is similarly affected.

Significant interactions with some antimicrobials can occur: erythromycin can reduce carbamazepine-10,11-epoxide levels by 40–60%, compromising seizure control in someone who, by definition, is already unwell. Interactions with antidepressants and antipsychotics (fluoxetine, fluvoxamine, paroxetine, trazodone, and olanzapine) make monitoring for neurotoxicity or worsening seizure control necessary.

Tips to aid adherence. Autoinduction during initial treatment will result in artificially high levels of carbamazepine. Children and parents should be warned about transient neurotoxic effects; slow titration regimens may help. Sustained-release formulations are preferable, both for improved tolerability and twice-daily rather than three-times-daily administration. Pharmacodynamic as well as pharmacokinetic interactions should be considered, particularly when co-administering with levetiracetam; it may be necessary to lower the dose of carbamazepine to avoid neurotoxicity.

Other considerations. A pretreatment screening test for HLA-B*1502 allele should be performed in individuals of Han Chinese or Thai origin (if positive, avoid the use of carbamazepine unless there is no alternative because of the risk of Stevens–Johnson syndrome).

Cenobamate[5]

Indications. Focal-onset seizures including focal to bilateral tonic-clonic seizures. Cenobamate is currently approved for use in adults only.

Off-label use. Recent studies have shown cenobamate to be effective in CYPWE.[6,7]

Mechanism of action. While the precise mechanism by which cenobamate exercises therapeutic effect is unknown, it is a positive allosteric modulator of subtypes of the GABA-A ion channel that does not bind to the benzodiazepine binding site. Cenobamate has also been shown to reduce repetitive neuronal firing by enhancing the inactivation of sodium channels and by inhibiting the persistent component of the sodium current.

Dose and administration. By mouth. Tablets (12.5 mg, 25 mg, 50 mg, 100 mg, 150 mg, 200 mg). Starting dose 12.5 mg od for 2 weeks, then 25 mg od for 2 weeks, then 50 mg od for 2 weeks, followed by further increments of 50 mg every 2 weeks; maintenance dose 200 mg od; maximum dose 400 mg od.

Contraindications. Familial short-QT syndrome.

Most common side effects. Somnolence, dizziness, fatigue, headache, and rash.

Significant interactions. Cenobamate raises plasma concentrations of phenytoin, phenobarbital, and clobazam's active metabolite N-desmethylclobazam, increasing the potential for adverse events. Careful therapeutic monitoring is required, and dose reductions may be needed. Cenobamate decreases plasma concentrations of lamotrigine and carbamazapine. Higher doses of cenobamate may be needed if co-administered with lamotrigine. Some patients may experience adverse effects at standard doses of carbamazepine and lamotrigine due to the pharmacodynamic effects of sodium channel blockers, in which case the dosage of these drugs may need to be reduced.

Adding cenobamate to cannabidiol or lacosamide may cause CNS dose-related adverse events such as sleepiness or dizziness, in which case the dosage of cannabidiol or lacosamide may need to be reduced. Reactive reductions of other ASM should be considered if neurotoxicity occurs.[8]

Cenobamate may also significantly reduce the efficacy of OCPs, thereby rendering them ineffective. Pharmacodynamic interactions between cenobamate and other CNS depressants, such as barbiturates, alcohol, and benzodiazepines, may lead to neurotoxicity.

Tips to aid adherence. Patients should be reviewed when the dosage of cenobamate has reached 100 mg/day to check for side effects as well as efficacy. Some patients may not need further dose escalation, and it is important to consider dose reduction of concomitant ASM as required (see Significant interactions above). If seizure control remains suboptimal after initiation of cenobamate, addition of a small dose of clobazam should be considered.[9]

Clobazam

Indications. Adjunctive treatment in epilepsy.

Off-label use. Children under 6 years old; monotherapy.

Mechanism of action. GABA agonist.

Dose and administration. By mouth. Tablets (10 mg), oral suspension (5 mg/5 mL and 10 mg/5 mL).

- 1 month to 5 years: starting dose 125 µg/kg bd, increasing according to response every 5 days; maintenance dose 250 µg/kg bd (maximum per dose 500 µg/kg bd); maximum dose 30 mg/day.
- 6–17 years: starting dose 5 mg/day, increasing if necessary at intervals of 5 days; maintenance dose 0.3–1 mg/kg/day depending on efficacy and tolerability and twice-daily dosing for doses exceeding 30 mg/day; maximum dose 60 mg/day.

Contraindications. Hyperkinesis, obsessional states, phobic states, and respiratory depression.

Cautions. Muscle weakness, organic brain changes, and personality disorder.

Most common side effects. Amnesia, ataxia, confusion, dependence, drowsiness the next day, lightheadedness the next day, muscle weakness, and paradoxical increase in aggression. Other side effects include dizziness, dysarthria, gastrointestinal disturbances, gynecomastia, incontinence, salivation changes, tremor, and visual disturbances.

Significant interactions. There is a low risk of interaction with enzyme-inducing ASM. Clobazam increases the risk of CNS depression when administered with other drugs with similar CNS side effects. This may affect the child's ability to perform skilled tasks. If awareness is impaired, young people should be advised not to drive (if they are eligible to learn to drive and/or have passed their driving test) or operate machinery. Young people should be informed that the effects of alcohol may also be increased and even be felt the next day.

Tips to aid adherence. If sedation occurs, patients should be advised to take a higher dose at night.

Other considerations. Short-term administration only is recommended for girls with catamenial epilepsy (CE) who experience cluster seizures around their menses and/or children (depending on individual circumstances) who experience an increase in seizures at times of illness/infection. A useful strategy to minimize seizures during this time is 10–20 mg/day (as per bodyweight) for up to 7–10 days. For CYPWE who regularly have clusters of seizures, a single dose of 10–30 mg (according to bodyweight) can have a useful prophylactic action if taken immediately after the first event. Care should be taken to ensure a prolonged period of weaning to prevent withdrawal side effects.

Clonazepam

Indications. All forms of epilepsy, in particular myoclonic seizures.

Mechanism of action. GABA agonist.

Dose and administration. By mouth. Tablets (0.5 mg, 1 mg, 2 mg), oral solution (500 µg/5 mL, 2 mg/5 mL).

- 1–11 months: starting dose 250 µg/night for 4 nights, increasing over 2–4 weeks to 0.5–1 mg/day, usually taken at night; may be given in 3 divided doses if necessary.
- 1–4 years: starting dose 250 µg/night for 4 nights, increasing over 2–4 weeks to 1–3 mg/day, usually taken at night; may be given in 3 divided doses if necessary.

- 5–11 years: starting dose 500 µg/night for 4 nights, increasing over 2–4 weeks to 3–6 mg/day, usually taken at night; may be given in 3 divided doses if necessary.
- 12–17 years: starting dose 1 mg/night for 4 nights, increasing over 2–4 weeks to 4–8 mg/day, usually taken at night; may be given in 3–4 divided doses if necessary.

Contraindications. Coma, current alcohol abuse, current drug abuse, and respiratory depression.

Most common side effects. Amnesia, bronchial hypersecretion in infants and small children, coordination disturbances, confusion, dependence, dizziness, drowsiness, fatigue, muscle hypotonia, nystagmus, poor concentration, restlessness, salivary hypersecretion in infants and small children, and withdrawal symptoms.

Significant interactions. There is a low risk of interaction with enzyme-inducing ASM. Clonazepam increases the risk of CNS depression when administered with other drugs with similar CNS side effects. This may affect the child's ability to perform skilled tasks. If awareness is impaired, young people should be advised not to drive (if they are eligible to learn to drive and/or they have passed their driving test) or operate machinery. Young people should be informed that the effects of alcohol may also be increased and may even be felt the next day.

Tips to aid adherence. If sedation occurs, patients should be advised to take a higher dose at night.

Diazepam

Indications. Status epilepticus (SE).

Mechanism of action. GABA agonist.

Dose and administration.

- By intravenous injection
  - Neonate: 300–400 µg/kg, then 300–400 µg/kg after 10 minutes if required, administered over 3–5 minutes.
  - 1 month to 11 years: 300–400 µg/kg (maximum per dose 10 mg), then 300–400 µg/kg after 10 minutes if required, administered over 3–5 minutes.
  - 12–17 years: 10 mg, then 10 mg after 10 minutes if required, administered over 3–5 minutes.

- By rectum
  - Neonate: 1.25–2.5 mg, then 1.25–2.5 mg after 5–10 minutes if required.
  - 1 month to 1 year: 5 mg, then 5 mg after 5–10 minutes if required.
  - 2–11 years: 5–10 mg, then 5–10 mg after 5–10 minutes if required.
  - 12–17 years: 10–20 mg, then 10–20 mg after 5–10 minutes if required.

Contraindications. CNS depression, compromised airway, hyperkinesia, obsessional states, phobic states, and respiratory depression. Injections containing benzyl alcohol should be avoided in neonates.

Cautions. Risk of venous thrombophlebitis with intravenous use, muscle weakness, organic brain changes, and parenteral administration.

Most common side effects. Amnesia, ataxia, confusion, dependence, drowsiness the next day, gastrointestinal disturbances, gynecomastia, incontinence, salivation changes, tremor, and visual disturbances.

Ethosuximide

Indications. Monotherapy for absence seizures, used as adjunctive treatment when monotherapy has failed. Also used as adjunctive treatment for atypical absence seizures and myoclonic seizures.

Mechanism of action. Binds to T-type voltage-sensitive channels.

Dose and administration. By mouth. Capsules (250 mg), oral solution (250 mg/5 mL).

- 1 month to 5 years: starting dose 5 mg/kg bd (maximum per dose 125 mg), increased every 5–7 days; maintenance dose 10–20 mg/kg bd (maximum per dose 500 mg); total daily dose may rarely be given in 3 divided doses.
- 6–17 years: starting dose 250 mg bd, increasing by 250 mg every 5–7 days according to response; maintenance dose 500–750 mg bd; maximum dose 1 g bd.

Contraindications. Acute porphyrias.

Most common side effects. Anorexia, abdominal pain, diarrhea, gastrointestinal disturbances, nausea, vomiting, and weight loss. Other side effects include aggression, ataxia, dizziness, drowsiness, euphoria, fatigue, headache, hiccups, impaired concentration, and irritability.

Significant interactions. Levels are often (but not always) increased by sodium valproate and reduced by carbamazepine, phenytoin, primidone, and phenobarbital, as well as lamotrigine: dose adjustment and/or plasma level monitoring may be required.

Other considerations. Ethosuximide is used for the control of absences. It should not be used to treat focal epilepsy.

Fosphenytoin is a pro-drug of phenytoin.

Indications. SE. Prophylaxis or treatment of seizures associated with neurosurgery or head injury. Temporary substitution for oral phenytoin (see page 99).

Mechanism of action. Phenytoin is believed to block sodium channels.

Dose and administration. By intravenous infusion in children aged 5–17 years. Solution for injection (750 mg/10 mL). Intermittent intravenous infusion given in glucose 5% or sodium chloride 0.9%; dilute to a concentration of 1.5–25 mg/mL.

- SE: starting dose 20 mg (phenytoin equivalent [PE])/kg, administered at 2–3 mg (PE)/kg/minute to a maximum of 150 mg (PE)/minute; maintenance dose 4–5 mg (PE)/kg/day in 1–4 divided doses, administered at 1–2 mg (PE)/kg/minute to a maximum of 100 mg (PE)/minute. Dose adjusted according to response and trough plasma-phenytoin concentration.
- Prophylaxis or treatment of seizures associated with neurosurgery or head injury: starting dose 10–15 mg (PE)/kg; maintenance dose 4–5 mg (PE)/kg/day in 1–4 divided doses, administered at 1–2 mg (PE)/kg/minute to a maximum of 100 mg (PE)/minute. Dose adjusted according to response and trough plasma-phenytoin concentration.
- Temporary substitution for oral phenytoin: same dose and dosing frequency as oral phenytoin therapy (see page 99), administered at 1–2 mg (PE)/kg/minute to a maximum of 100 mg (PE)/minute. Dose adjusted according to response and trough plasma-phenytoin concentration.

Contraindications. Acute porphyria, second-degree heart block, sinoatrial block, sinus bradycardia, Stokes–Adams syndrome, third-degree heart block.

Cautions. Heart failure, hypotension, injection solutions (irritant to tissues), and respiratory depression. Resuscitation facilities must be available.

Most common side effects. Alterations in respiratory function, arrhythmias, asthenia, cardiovascular collapse (particularly if injection is too rapid), chills, CNS depression (particularly if injection is too rapid), dry mouth, dysarthria, ecchymosis, euphoria, hypotension, incoordination, pruritus, respiratory arrest, taste disturbance, tinnitus, vasodilatation, and visual disturbance.

Cardiovascular reactions. Intravenous infusion of fosphenytoin has been associated with severe cardiovascular reactions including asystole, ventricular fibrillation, and cardiac arrest. Hypotension, bradycardia, and heart block have also been reported.

Gabapentin

Indications. Monotherapy and adjunctive treatment for focal-onset seizures with or without bilateral tonic-clonic seizures.

Off-label use. Children under 6 years old. Doses over 50 mg/kg/day in children under 12 years old.

Mechanism of action. Mimics the neurotransmitter GABA but does not bind to GABA receptors. It is likely to involve the inhibition of the $\alpha2$-δ subunit of calcium channels.

Dose and administration. By mouth. Tablets (600 mg, 800 mg), capsules (100 mg, 300 mg, 400 mg), oral solution (50 mg/mL, 250 mg/5 mL).

- Adjunctive treatment
  - 2–5 years: starting dose 10 mg/kg/day on day 1, 10 mg/kg bd on day 2, 10 mg/kg tid on day 3, increasing to 30–70 mg/kg/day in 3 divided doses, adjusted according to response. Some children may not tolerate daily increments in which case longer intervals (up to weekly) may be more appropriate.
  - 6–11 years: starting dose 10 mg/kg/day (maximum per dose 300 mg) on day 1, 10 mg/kg bd (maximum per dose 300 mg) on day 2, 10 mg/kg tid (maximum per dose 300 mg) on day 3; maintenance dose 25–35 mg/kg/day in 3 divided doses. Some children may not tolerate daily increments in which case longer intervals (up to weekly) may be more appropriate; maximum dose 70 mg/kg/day.
  - 12–17 years: starting dose 300 mg/day on day 1, 300 mg bd on day 2, 300 mg tid on day 3; alternatively, a starting dose of 300 mg tid on day 1, increasing by 300 mg every 2–3 days in 3 divided doses, adjusted according to response; maintenance dose 0.9–3.6 g/day in 3 divided doses (maximum per dose 1.6 g tid).

Some children may not tolerate daily increments in which case longer intervals (up to weekly) may be more appropriate.

- Monotherapy
  - 12–17 years: starting dose 300 mg/day on day 1, 300 mg bd on day 2, 300 mg tid on day 3; alternatively, a starting dose of 300 mg tid on day 1, increasing by 300 mg every 2–3 days in 3 divided doses, adjusted according to response; maintenance dose 0.9–3.6 g/day in 3 divided doses (maximum per dose 1.6 g tid). Some children may not tolerate daily increments in which case longer intervals (up to weekly) may be more appropriate.

Contraindications. Diabetes mellitus, high doses of oral solution in adolescents with low bodyweight, and history of psychotic illness and mixed seizures (including absences).

Most common side effects. Abdominal pain, abnormal reflexes, abnormal thoughts, acne, amnesia, anorexia, anxiety, arthralgia, ataxia, confusion, constipation, convulsions, cough, depression, diarrhea, dizziness, drowsiness, dry mouth, dry throat, dyspepsia, dyspnea, edema, emotional lability, fever, flatulence, flu syndrome, gingivitis, headache, hostility, hypertension, impotence, increased appetite, insomnia, leucopenia, malaise, movement disorders, myalgia, nausea, nervousness, nystagmus, paresthesia, pruritus, rash, rhinitis, speech disorder, tremor, twitching, vasodilatation, vertigo, visual disturbance, vomiting, and weight loss.

Significant interactions. There is a rare risk of severe respiratory depression when gabapentin is used in combination with opioid medicines and other CNS depressants.

Tips to aid adherence. Use 1–2 weekly titration rates, rather than 1–3 days, along with lower starting doses.

Other considerations. In the UK, gabapentin is classified as a Class C controlled substance and a Schedule 3 drug because of concerns about abuse. In the USA, gabapentin is not a federally controlled substance, but it is a Schedule V controlled drug in some states. Any history of drug abuse should be determined before prescribing and the patient should be observed for signs of abuse and dependence. High doses of the oral solution should be used with caution in patients with diabetes mellitus or low bodyweight, as levels of propylene glycol, acesulfame K, and saccharin sodium are high.

Lacosamide

Indications. Monotherapy and adjunctive treatment for focal-onset seizures with or without bilateral tonic-clonic seizures.

Mechanism of action. Enhances the number of sodium channels entering the slow inactivated state.

Dose and administration. By mouth or intravenous infusion. Tablets (50 mg, 100 mg, 150 mg, 200 mg), oral solution (10 mg/mL), solution for infusion (200 mg/20 mL).

- Monotherapy
  - 2–17 years (bodyweight ≥50 kg): starting dose 50 mg bd, increasing to 100 mg bd after 1 week (alternative starting dose 100 mg bd). Increase at weekly intervals by 50 mg bd if necessary and tolerated (maximum per dose 300 mg bd).
  - 2–17 years (bodyweight <50 kg): starting dose 1 mg/kg bd, increasing to 2 mg/kg bd after 1 week. Increase at weekly intervals by 1 mg/kg bd if necessary and tolerated (maximum per dose 6 mg/kg bd for bodyweight 10–39 kg, or 5 mg/kg bd for bodyweight 40–49 kg).
- Adjunctive treatment
  - 2–17 years (bodyweight ≥50 kg): starting dose 50 mg bd, increasing to 100 mg bd after 1 week, increasing in weekly intervals by 50 mg bd if necessary and tolerated (maximum per dose 200 mg bd).
  - 2–17 years (bodyweight <50 kg): starting dose 1 mg/kg bd, increasing to 2 mg/kg bd after 1 week. Increase at weekly intervals by 1 mg/kg bd if necessary and tolerated (maximum per dose 6 mg/kg bd for bodyweight 10–19 kg, 5 mg/kg bd for bodyweight 20–29 kg, or 4 mg/kg bd for bodyweight 30–49 kg).
- Alternative loading (both as monotherapy or adjunctive therapy) under close medical supervision can be given to children of bodyweight 50 kg and above when rapid therapeutic plasma concentrations are needed. This comprises a starting dose of 200 mg, followed by 100 mg bd every 12 hours, increasing at weekly intervals by 50 mg bd if necessary and tolerated (maximum per dose 300 mg bd for monotherapy, or 200 mg bd for adjunctive therapy).

Contraindications. Second- or third-degree AV block.

Cautions. Conduction problems, risk of prolonged PR interval (onset of P wave to start of QRS complex), and severe cardiac disease. Patients must have an ECG before treatment and caution should be applied if other medicinal products associated with PR prolongation are being taken.

Most common side effects. Abnormal gait, blurred vision, cognitive disorder, constipation, depression, dizziness, drowsiness, fatigue, flatulence, headache, impaired coordination, nausea, nystagmus, pruritus, tremor, and vomiting.

Significant interactions. Phenytoin, phenobarbital, and carbamazepine may reduce lacosamide concentrations.

Tips to aid adherence. Lacosamide should be titrated slowly, starting at 50 mg at night for 2 weeks, increasing to 50 mg bd.

Lamotrigine

Indications. Monotherapy and adjunctive treatment for focal-onset seizures with or without bilateral tonic-clonic seizures, GTCS, and seizures associated with LGS. Monotherapy of typical absence seizures.

Mechanism of action. Inhibits sodium currents by selectively binding to inactivated sodium channels, suppressing the release of glutamate.

Dose and administration. By mouth. Tablets (25 mg, 50 mg, 100 mg, 200 mg), dispersible tablets (2 mg, 5 mg, 25 mg, 100 mg). Dose titration should be repeated if restarting after more than 5 days without medication.

- Monotherapy of focal seizures, GTCS, and LGS (12–17 years): starting dose 25 mg/day for 2 weeks, then 50 mg/day for 2 weeks, then increase by up to 100 mg every 1–2 weeks according to response; maintenance dose 100–200 mg/day in 1–2 divided doses; maximum dose 500 mg/day.
- Monotherapy of typical absence seizures (2–11 years): starting dose 300 µg/kg/day in 1–2 divided doses for 2 weeks, then 600 µg/kg/day in 1–2 divided doses for 2 weeks, then increase by up to 600 µg/kg every 1–2 weeks; maintenance dose 1–10 mg/kg/day in 1–2 divided doses; maximum dose 15 mg/kg/day.
- Adjunctive treatment of focal seizures, GTCS, and LGS with sodium valproate

- 2–11 years (bodyweight < 13 kg): starting dose 2 mg od on alternate days for 2 weeks, then 300 µg/kg/day for 2 weeks, then increase by up to 300 µg/kg every 1–2 weeks according to response; maintenance dose 1–5 mg/kg/day in 1–2 divided doses; maximum dose 200 mg/day.
- 2–11 years (bodyweight ≥ 13 kg): starting dose 150 µg/kg/day for 2 weeks, then 300 µg/kg/day for 2 weeks, then increase by up to 300 µg/kg every 1–2 weeks; maintenance dose 1–5 mg/kg/day in 1–2 divided doses; maximum dose 200 mg/day.
- 12–17 years: starting dose 25 mg od on alternate days for 2 weeks, then 25 mg/day for 2 weeks, then increase by up to 50 mg every 1–2 weeks; maintenance dose 100–200 mg/day in 1–2 divided doses.
• Adjunctive treatment of focal seizures, GTCS, and LGS (with enzyme-inducing drugs) without sodium valproate
  - 2–11 years: starting dose 300 µg/kg bd for 2 weeks, then 600 µg/kg bd for 2 weeks, then increase by up to 1.2 mg/kg every 1–2 weeks; maintenance dose 5–15 mg/kg/day in 1–2 divided doses; maximum dose 400 mg/day.
  - 12–17 years: starting dose 50 mg/day for 2 weeks, then 50 mg bd for 2 weeks, then increase by up to 100 mg every 1–2 weeks; maintenance dose 200–400 mg/day in 2 divided doses; maximum dose 700 mg/day.
• Adjunctive treatment of focal seizures, GTCS, and LGS (without enzyme-inducing drugs) without sodium valproate
  - 2–11 years: starting dose 300 µg/kg/day in 1–2 divided doses for 2 weeks, then 600 µg/kg/day in 1–2 divided doses for 2 weeks, then increase by up to 600 µg/kg every 1–2 weeks; maintenance dose 1–10 mg/kg/day in 1–2 divided doses; maximum dose 200 mg/day.
  - 12–17 years: starting dose 25 mg/day for 2 weeks, then 50 mg/day for 2 weeks, then increase by up to 100 mg every 1–2 weeks; maintenance dose 100–200 mg/day in 1–2 divided doses.

Cautions. Myoclonic seizures, as lamotrigine can make myoclonus worsen.

Most common side effects. Blurred vision, aggression, agitation, arthralgia, ataxia, back pain, dry mouth, headache, insomnia, nausea, nystagmus, rash, tremor, and vomiting.

Significant interactions. When used as monotherapy, the half-life of lamotrigine is approximately 24 hours. When given to patients already being treated with carbamazepine, phenytoin, or phenobarbital the half-life falls to about 15 hours. Sodium valproate inhibits glucuronidation of lamotrigine, prolonging its half-life to around 60 hours. Withdrawal of enzyme-inducing ASM therefore causes a rise in the circulating concentrations of lamotrigine, while discontinuing sodium valproate produces a fall. Neurotoxicity (headache, dizziness, nausea, diplopia, ataxia) is common when lamotrigine is introduced in patients established on high-dose carbamazepine or oxcarbazepine, so doses of carbamazepine or oxcarbazepine should be given 2–3 hours apart from lamotrigine. A pharmacodynamic interaction may also explain the marked tremor seen in some patients taking sodium valproate and lamotrigine in combination.

In combination with the OCP, lamotrigine levels can fall by over 50%. Dose adjustment may be required. In practice, this can be problematic because of the 'pill-free week' when lamotrigine concentrations would be significantly higher, possibly resulting in neurotoxicity. Lamotrigine also reduces progesterone levels by about 20%, but this is not thought to result in ovulation.

Rifampicin, lopinavir, ritonavir, and atanzavir can reduce plasma concentrations of lamotrigine: dose adjustments may be required.

Tips to aid adherence. Patients who have vivid dreams/sleep disturbances should be advised to take their night-time dose earlier. Slower titration is recommended when adding lamotrigine to sodium valproate: smaller doses are available in dispersible form.

Other considerations. Serum concentrations of lamotrigine fall during pregnancy: concentrations should be monitored and doses adjusted accordingly.

Levetiracetam

Indications. Monotherapy and adjunctive treatment for focal-onset seizures with or without bilateral tonic-clonic seizures. Adjunctive treatment of myoclonic seizures and tonic-clonic seizures.

Off-label use. Granules are not licensed for use in children under 6 years, for initial treatment in children with bodyweight under 25 kg, or for doses below 250 mg. Levetiracetam is used intravenously for the treatment of convulsive SE (intravenous infusion of 40 mg/kg, administered with expert advice as a single dose and according to local protocols) but it is not licensed for this indication.

Mechanism of action. SV2A ligand.

Dose and administration. By mouth or intravenous infusion. Tablets (250 mg, 500 mg, 750 mg, 1000 mg), granules (250 mg, 500 mg, 1000 mg), oral solution (100 mg/mL), solution for infusion (500 mg/5 mL).

- Monotherapy (16–17 years, by mouth or intravenous infusion): starting dose 250 mg/day for 1 week, then 250 mg bd, then increase every 2 weeks by 250 mg bd adjusted according to response (maximum per dose 1.5 g bd).
- Adjunctive oral treatment of focal-onset seizures with or without bilateral tonic-clonic seizures
  - 1–5 months: starting dose 7 mg/kg/day, increasing every 2 weeks by up to 7 mg/kg bd (maximum per dose 21 mg/kg bd).
  - 6 months to 17 years (bodyweight < 50 kg): starting dose 10 mg/kg/day, increasing every 2 weeks by up to 10 mg/kg bd (maximum per dose 30 mg/kg bd).
  - 12–17 years (bodyweight ≥ 50 kg): starting dose 250 mg bd, increasing every 2–4 weeks by 500 mg bd (maximum per dose 1.5 g bd).
- Adjunctive intravenous infusion for focal-onset seizures with or without bilateral tonic-clonic seizures
  - 4–17 years (bodyweight < 50 kg): starting dose 10 mg/kg/day, increasing by up to 10 mg/kg bd every 2 weeks (maximum per dose 30 mg/kg bd).
  - 12–17 years (bodyweight ≥ 50 kg): starting dose 250 mg bd, increasing by 500 mg bd every 2 weeks (maximum per dose 1.5 g bd).
- Adjunctive treatment (by mouth or intravenous infusion) of myoclonic seizures and tonic-clonic seizures
  - 12–17 years (bodyweight < 50 kg): starting dose 10 mg/kg/day, increasing by up to 10 mg/kg bd every 2 weeks (maximum per dose 30 mg/kg bd).
  - 12–17 years (bodyweight ≥ 50 kg): starting dose 250 mg bd increasing by 500 mg bd every 2 weeks (maximum per dose 1.5 g bd).

Most common side effects. Abdominal pain, aggression, anorexia, anxiety, ataxia, convulsion, cough, nasopharyngitis, nausea, rash, tremor, vertigo, and vomiting.

Significant interactions. Levetiracetam decreases the clearance of methotrexate: both levetiracetam and methotrexate concentrations should be monitored.

Tips to aid adherence. Slower titration reduces the risk of behavioral side effects. In addition, pyridoxine (vitamin B6), 50–200 mg/day, helps to alleviate mood-related side effects, though many of the studies in this area are not robust.

Lorazepam

Indications. SE.

Off-label use. Treatment of febrile convulsions.

Mechanism of action. Binds to receptors on the postsynaptic GABA-A ligand-gated chloride channel neuron at several sites within the CNS and enhances the inhibitory effect of GABA.

Dose and administration. By slow intravenous infusion into a large vein.

- Neonate: first dose 100 µg/kg; second dose 100 µg/kg, administered after 5–10 minutes if first dose is ineffective.
- 1 month to 11 years: first dose 100 µg/kg (maximum per dose 4 mg); second dose 100 µg/kg (maximum per dose 4 mg) administered after 5–10 minutes if first dose is ineffective.
- 12–17 years: first dose 4 mg; second dose 4 mg, administered after 5–10 minutes if first dose is ineffective.

Contraindications. CNS depression, compromised airway, hyperkinesia, obsessional states, phobic states, and respiratory depression. Injections containing benzyl alcohol should be avoided in neonates.

Most common side effects. Amnesia, ataxia, confusion, dependence, drowsiness the next day, lightheadedness the next day, muscle weakness, and a paradoxical increase in aggression.

Midazolam

Indications. SE and febrile convulsions.

Mechanism of action. GABA agonist.

Dose and administration. Oromucosal administration or by intravenous injection and continuous intravenous infusion. Oromucosal solution (2.5 mg/0.25 or 0.5 mL, 5 mg/0.5 or 1 mL, 7.5 mg/0.75 or 1.5 mL, 10 mg/1 or 2 mL), oral solution (2 mg/mL, 5 mg/mL), solution for injection (2 mg/2 mL, 5 mg/5 mL, 10 mg/5 mL, 10 mg/2 mL, 15 mg/3 mL, 50 mg/10 mL), solution for infusion (50 or 100 mg/50 mL).

- Oromucosal administration
  - Neonate: 300 µg/kg, then 300 µg/kg after 5–10 minutes if required.
  - 1–2 months: 300 µg/kg (maximum per dose 2.5 mg), then 300 µg/kg after 5–10 minutes (maximum per dose 2.5 mg) if required.
  - 3–11 months: 2.5 mg, then 2.5 mg after 5–10 minutes if required.
  - 1–4 years: 5 mg, then 5 mg after 5–10 minutes if required.
  - 5–9 years: 7.5 mg, then 7.5 mg after 5–10 minutes if required.
  - 10–17 years: 10 mg, then 10 mg after 5–10 minutes if required.
- Intravenous injection and continuous infusion
  - Neonate to 17 years: 150–200 µg/kg by intravenous injection, then 60 µg/kg/hour by continuous intravenous infusion, increasing by 60 µg/kg/hour every 15 minutes (maximum per dose 300 µg/kg/hour) until seizure controlled.

Contraindications. CNS and respiratory depression in patients whose airways are compromised.

Most common side effects. Respiratory depression, hypotension, and sedation.

Significant interactions. There is a low risk of interaction with enzyme-inducing ASM. Midazolam increases the risk of CNS depression when administered with other drugs with similar CNS side effects, which may affect the patient's ability to perform skilled tasks.

Other considerations. See Chapter 9 on management of seizures in a community setting and the training requirements for family members and caregivers.

Oxcarbazepine

Indications. Monotherapy or adjunctive treatment for focal-onset seizures with or without bilateral tonic-clonic seizures.

Mechanism of action. Sodium channel blocker. Oxcarbazepine also modulates calcium and potassium currents.

Dose and administration. By mouth. Tablets (150 mg, 300 mg, 600 mg), oral suspension (60 mg/mL).

- 6–17 years: starting dose 4–5 mg/kg bd (maximum per dose 300 mg), increasing by up to 5 mg/kg bd at weekly intervals according to response; maintenance dose (adjunctive therapy) 15 mg/kg bd; maximum dose 46 mg/kg/day.

Contraindications. Acute porphyrias, cardiac conduction disorders, heart failure, and hyponatremia.

Most common side effects. CNS side effects, including drowsiness, dizziness, headache, diplopia, nausea, vomiting, and ataxia. Other side effects include depression, mood changes, cognitive impairment, hyponatremia, and rash (less frequently than with carbamazepine).

Significant interactions. Interactions are similar to those with carbamazepine, but oxcarbazepine is a less potent enzyme inducer so the interactions, and therefore the implications for treatment, are less marked. It reduces the effect of the OCP.

Tips to aid adherence. If a twice-daily dose cannot be tolerated, oxcarbazepine can be taken three times a day.

Other considerations. Plasma sodium concentration should be regularly tested in patients at risk of hyponatremia. Bodyweight should be monitored in patients with heart failure. It is also important to be aware that oxcarbazepine may exacerbate absence and myoclonic seizures.

A pretreatment screening test for HLA-B*1502 allele should be performed in individuals of Han Chinese or Thai origin (if it is positive, oxcarbazepine should not be administered unless there is no alternative because of the risk of Stevens–Johnson syndrome).

Paraldehyde

Indications. SE.

Mechanism of action. The exact mechanism of action is unknown. It is thought to reduce the release of acetylcholine in response to neuronal depolarization.

Dose and administration. By rectum. Premixed solution of paraldehyde in an equal volume of olive oil. One dose of 0.8 mL/kg (maximum per dose 20 mL).

Contraindications. Gastric disorders. Rectal administration should be avoided in patients with colitis.

Most common side effects. Rash.

Other considerations. Once drawn up into a syringe, the solution must be administered within 15 minutes, otherwise the paraldehyde will start to eat into the plastic syringe.

Perampanel

Indications. Adjunctive treatment for focal-onset seizures with or without bilateral tonic-clonic seizures, and for GTCS.

Mechanism of action. A unique, highly selective, non-competitive antagonist of the ionotropic α-amino-3-hydroxy-5-methyl-4-isoxazole propionic acid (AMPA) glutamate receptor on postsynaptic neurons. Activation of AMPA receptors by glutamate is thought to be responsible for most fast excitatory synaptic transmission in the brain. However, the precise mechanism of action is not fully known.

Dose and administration. By mouth. Tablets (2 mg, 4 mg, 6 mg, 8 mg, 10 mg, 12 mg), oral suspension (0.5 mg/mL).

- 4–11 years: starting dose 1 mg/day (if bodyweight ≤29 kg) or 2 mg/day (if bodyweight ≥30 kg) taken at bedtime, increasing by 1 mg or 2 mg, respectively, at least every 2 weeks according to response; maintenance dose 2–4 mg/day (if bodyweight <20 kg), 4–6 mg/day (if bodyweight 20–29 kg), or 4–8 mg/day (if bodyweight ≥30 kg); maximum dose 6 mg/day, 8 mg/day, or 12 mg/day, respectively.
- 12–17 years: starting dose 2 mg/day taken at bedtime, increasing by 2 mg at least every 2 weeks according to response; maintenance dose 4–8 mg/day; maximum dose 12 mg/day.

Contraindications. None, but perampanel should be avoided in patients with severe hepatic and renal impairment.

Most common side effects. Dizziness, somnolence, nausea, diplopia, ataxia, vertigo, headache, decreased and increased appetite, fatigue, gait disturbance, and falls. Psychiatric disorders such as aggression, anger, anxiety, and confusion are not uncommon.

Significant interactions. Phenytoin, carbamazepine, and oxcarbazepine decrease levels of perampanel: doses should be adjusted as necessary. In particular, carbamazepine increases perampanel clearance by up to threefold. Perampanel does not seem to affect the metabolism of other ASM. At high doses, perampanel decreases levanorgestrol but not ethinylestradiol exposure. There is a possibility of decreased efficacy of progesterone-containing oral contraceptives in women taking perampanel, 12 mg/day.

Tips to aid adherence. Slow titration rates are vital. In the authors' experience, a starting dose of 2 mg/day should be increased to 4 mg/day after 4 weeks, with titration continuing no faster than 4 mg every 4 weeks until seizure control is established. For some people, particularly those with intellectual disability (ID), even slower regimens should be implemented. Given the drug's half-life of around 120 hours, it is feasible to start the drug at 2 mg once every other day or even once every 3 days to alleviate side effects. It is very important to give perampanel at bedtime to avoid the neurotoxicity associated with peak plasma concentrations.

Other considerations. Perampanel has by far the longest half-life of any ASM. This may make it particularly helpful for people who find it difficult to remember to take medication.

Phenobarbital

Indications. All forms of epilepsy except for typical absence seizures. Also, SE.

Mechanism of action. GABA agonist.

Dose and administration. By mouth or slow intravenous injection. Tablets (15 mg, 30 mg, 60 mg), ethanol-free oral solution (50 mg/5 mL), solution for injection (30 mg/mL, 60 mg/mL, 200 mg/mL).

- Neonate: initially 20 mg/kg (by slow intravenous injection), then (by mouth or slow intravenous injection) 2.5–5 mg/kg/day, adjusted according to response. For SE (by slow intravenous injection), initially 20 mg/kg, then 2.5–5 mg/kg od or bd.
- 1 month to 11 years: initially 1–1.5 mg/kg bd (by mouth), increasing by 2 mg/kg/day as required; maintenance dose 2.5–4 mg/kg od or bd. For SE (by slow intravenous injection), initially 20 mg/kg, then 2.5–5 mg/kg od or bd.
- 12–17 years: 60–180 mg/day (by mouth). For SE (by slow intravenous injection), initially 20 mg/kg (maximum per dose 1 g), then 300 mg bd.

Contraindications. Acute porphyrias. Phenobarbital should be avoided in young people with a history of drug and alcohol abuse or respiratory depression, as it can cause CNS-depressant effects.

Most common side effects. Sedation and behavioral problems, such as anxiety, depression, and agitation. Other side effects include cognitive impairment, memory loss, risk of allergic rash, osteoporosis, folate deficiency, and Dupuytren's contracture.

Significant interactions. Oxcarbazepine, phenytoin, and sodium valproate increase phenobarbital plasma concentrations. Patients being treated concomitantly with sodium valproate should be monitored for signs of hyperammonemia (half of reported cases are asymptomatic and do not necessarily result in clinical encephalopathy). Vigabatrin possibly decreases phenobarbital plasma concentrations. Phenobarbital is a powerful inducer of hepatic metabolism, accelerating the clearance of many other lipid-soluble drugs. It renders the OCP ineffective.

Tips to aid adherence. Patients who cannot tolerate one daily dose may take phenobarbital in 2–3 divided doses.

Other considerations. Phenobarbital is no longer considered first-line treatment (except for neonatal seizures) because of its significant side effects and many clinically relevant interactions. However, people who have been taking phenobarbital for many years without problems should be advised to remain on it rather than switching to a newer ASM. It still has a role in drug-resistant epilepsy and is cheap and therefore readily available in developing economies.

Phenobarbital Elixir BP (15 mg/5 mL) contains 38% v/v of ethanol and should be avoided in children.

Phenytoin

Indications. Focal-onset seizures and tonic-clonic seizures. It can also be given during and after neurosurgery or severe head injury to prevent and treat seizures. Also, SE.

Mechanism of action. Sodium channel blocker.

Dose and administration. By mouth or slow intravenous injection or intravenous infusion. Tablets (100 mg), chewable tablets (50 mg), capsules (25 mg, 50 mg, 100 mg, 300 mg), oral suspension (30 mg/5 mL), solution for injection (250 mg/5 mL).

* Focal-onset and tonic-clonic seizures
  – Neonate: initial loading dose 18 mg/kg, administered over 20–30 minutes by slow intravenous injection, then oral 2.5–5 mg/kg bd adjusted according to response and plasma-phenytoin concentration (maximum per dose 7.5 mg/kg bd).

- 1 month to 11 years: oral starting dose 1.5–2.5 mg/kg bd, then increase according to therapeutic response and plasma-phenytoin concentration to 2.5–5 mg/kg bd (maximum per dose 7.5 mg/kg bd); maximum dose 300 mg/day.
- 12–17 years: oral starting dose 75–150 mg bd, then increase according to therapeutic response and plasma-phenytoin concentration to 150–200 mg bd (maximum per dose 300 mg bd).
- Prevention and treatment of seizures during or following neurosurgery or severe head injury
  - Child: oral starting dose 2.5 mg/kg bd, then increase according to therapeutic response and plasma-phenytoin concentration to 4–8 mg/kg/day; maximum dose 300 mg/day.
- SE (by slow intravenous injection or infusion)
  - Neonate to 11 years: loading dose 20 mg/kg, then 2.5–5 mg/kg bd.
  - 12–17 years: loading dose 20 mg/kg, then up to 100 mg tid or qid.

Contraindications. Acute porphyrias, sinus bradycardia, second- and third-degree heart block, and Adams–Stokes syndrome.

Most common side effects. Neurotoxic symptoms (ataxia, nystagmus, dysarthria, asterixis, somnolence) typically present 8–12 hours after an oral dose. Chronic dysmorphic effects (gingival hyperplasia, hirsutism, acne, facial coarsening) occur after months of treatment.

Significant interactions. Phenytoin reduces the serum concentrations of carbamazepine, sodium valproate, lamotrigine, perampanel, and topiramate. Phenytoin is tightly bound to circulating albumin and may be displaced by other drugs; some of these, such as sodium valproate, also inhibit the metabolism of phenytoin. Phenytoin's induction of hepatic enzymes may also reduce the effectiveness of other lipid-soluble drugs, including oral contraceptives and anticoagulants.

Tips to aid adherence. Patients with erratic adherence should be treated twice daily to lessen the effect of a missed dose.

Other considerations. Phenytoin has non-linear pharmacokinetics, so small dose adjustments can have large effects on plasma concentrations. Plasma levels should be assessed after dose changes and treatment with concomitant drugs that interact, and routinely every 12 months. Plasma levels will guide dosage.

Care should be taken when switching between brands, as preparations containing phenytoin sodium are not equivalent to those containing phenytoin base. Phenytoin may exacerbate absence and myoclonic seizures. A pretreatment screening test for HLA-B*1502 allele should be performed in individuals of Han Chinese or Thai origin (if it is positive, phenytoin should not be administered unless it is essential, because of the increased risk of Stevens–Johnson syndrome in the presence of the HLA-B*1502 allele).

Primidone

Indications. All forms of epilepsy except typical absence seizures.

Mechanism of action. Not fully understood; however, it is metabolized in the liver to phenobarbital and another active substance, phenylethylmalonamide.

Dose and administration. By mouth. Tablets (50 mg, 250 mg), oral suspension (125 mg/5 mL).

- 1 month to 8 years: starting dose 125 mg at night, increasing by 125 mg every 3 days according to response; maintenance dose 125–250 mg bd (1 month to 1 year), 250–375 mg bd (2–4 years), 375–500 mg bd (5–8 years).
- 9–17 years: starting dose 125 mg at night, increasing by 125 mg every 3 days to 250 mg bd, then increasing by 250 mg every 3 days (maximum per dose 750 mg bd) according to response.

Contraindications. Acute porphyrias. Also, caution should be applied in young people with a history of drug and alcohol abuse or respiratory depression, as primidone can cause CNS depressant effects.

Most common side effects. Ataxia, dizziness, nausea, and visual impairment.

Significant interactions. It is advisable to consult national product labeling before prescribing concomitant treatment with primidone because of the very large number of clinically relevant interactions. It should also be noted that primidone is metabolized to phenobarbital (see page 98).

Primidone raises metabolism and thereby may decrease plasma concentrations of carbamazepine, lamotrigine, oxcarbazepine (which itself raises metabolism and may reduce plasma levels of primidone), perampanel, phenytoin (which itself raises phenobarbital concentrations resulting in possible toxicity; patients taking phenytoin may experience toxicity when they stop primidone), stiripentol, tiagabine, sodium valproate, and zonisamide.

Primidone reduces the effect of the OCP. Isoniazid and nicotinamide cause very high levels of primidone, with neurotoxic side effects.

Tips to aid adherence. Clinicians should be extremely mindful of drug interactions, particularly if phenytoin or carbamazepine are added to pre-existing primidone therapy. This can raise therapeutic levels to toxic levels. In addition, acute adverse reactions can occur in the early stages of treatment and much slower titration regimens are advised in clinical practice than in published formularies.

Other considerations. Rather like phenobarbital, primidone is no longer considered a first-line ASM. However, if a patient has been stable on the drug for many years, it may be better to maintain treatment than switch to a newer ASM. The half-life of primidone is short (3.3–11 hours), so dosing three times a day may be appropriate, though in clinical practice a twice-daily regimen is usually preferred.

Rufinamide

Indications. Adjunctive treatment for seizures associated with LGS.

Mechanism of action. Rufinamide is a triazole derivative that reduces the recovery capacity of neuronal sodium channels after inactivation, thereby limiting action potential firing. Other unknown mechanisms of action are also likely given the drug's broad spectrum of antiseizure properties.

Dose and administration. By mouth. Tablets (100 mg, 200 mg, 400 mg), oral suspension (40 mg/mL, may contain propylene glycol). Rufinamide should be initiated by a specialist.

- 1–3 years: starting dose 5 mg/kg bd, increasing not less than every 3 days by up to 5 mg/kg bd according to response to target (maximum) dose. Maximum per dose 22.5 mg/kg bd (without sodium valproate) or 15 mg/kg bd (with sodium valproate); each dose should be given to the nearest 0.5 mL.
- 4–17 years (bodyweight <30 kg): starting dose 100 mg bd, increasing not less than every 3 days (without valproate) or not less than every 2 days (with valproate) by 100 mg bd according to response. Maximum per dose 500 mg bd (without valproate), 300 mg bd (with valproate).
- 4–17 years (bodyweight 30–50 kg): starting dose 200 mg bd, increasing not less than every 2 days by 200 mg bd according to

response. Maximum per dose 900 mg bd (without valproate),
600 mg bd (with valproate).

- 4–17 years (bodyweight 50.1–70 kg): starting dose 200 mg bd,
  increasing not less than every 2 days by 200 mg bd according to
  response. Maximum per dose 1.2 g bd (without valproate),
  800 mg bd (with valproate).
- 4–17 years (bodyweight ≥70.1 kg): starting dose 200 mg bd,
  increasing not less than every 2 days by 200 mg bd according to
  response. Maximum per dose 1.6 g bd (without valproate), 1.1 g bd
  (with valproate).

Contraindications. Patients who are at risk of shortening of
QTc interval.

Most common side effects. Headache, dizziness, fatigue, and
somnolence.

Significant interactions. Sodium valproate can significantly
increase rufinamide plasma levels. Rufinamide may reduce the
clearance of phenytoin, hence increasing circulating concentrations of
phenytoin. It also induces the metabolism of the ethinylestradiol and
norethisterone combined OCP.

Tips to aid adherence. Tablets can be crushed and swallowed with
water.

Other considerations. Rufinamide has 'orphan drug' status for LGS
because it is particularly effective against tonic and atonic seizures.
Both seizure types can cause devastating falls and injuries, so while
other ASM may be required, rufinamide can be an effective adjunct in
patients with the syndrome.

Sodium valproate

Indications. All forms of epilepsy, especially genetic generalized
epilepsy (GGE). Also, SE.

Mechanism of action. Limits sustained repetitive firing by a use- and
voltage-dependent effect on sodium channels and calcium channels.
It also facilitates the effects of the inhibitory neurotransmitter GABA
and N-methyl D-aspartate (NMDA) receptor antagonism.

Dose and administration. By mouth using immediate-release
medicines or by intravenous injection or infusion. Tablets (100 mg),
modified-release tablets (200 mg, 300 mg, 500 mg), gastroresistant
tablets (200 mg, 500 mg), modified-release capsules (150 mg, 300 mg),

modified-release granules (50 mg, 100 mg, 250 mg, 500 mg, 750 mg, 1000 mg), oral solution (200 mg/5 mL), solution for injection (300 mg/3 mL, 400 mg/4 mL), powder and solvent for solution for injection (400 mg). Clinical chemistry and hematologic parameters should be monitored if the dose exceeds 40 mg/kg/day.

- By mouth or by rectum
  - Neonate: starting dose 20 mg/kg/day; maintenance dose 10 mg/kg bd.
  - 1 month to 11 years: starting dose 10–15 mg/kg/day in 1–2 divided doses (maximum per dose 600 mg); maintenance dose 25–30 mg/kg/day in 2 divided doses. Up to 60 mg/kg/day may be used in 2 divided doses for infantile spasms.
  - 12–17 years: starting dose 600 mg/day in 1–2 divided doses, increasing every 3 days by 150–300 mg; maintenance dose 1–2 g/day in 2 divided doses; maximum dose 2.5 g/day.
- By intravenous injection or infusion, or continuous infusion
  - Neonate: 10 mg/kg bd (by intravenous injection).
  - 1 month to 11 years: starting dose by intravenous injection 10 mg/kg, increasing to 20–40 mg/kg/day in 2–4 divided doses by intravenous infusion or injection; alternatively, increasing to 20–40 mg/kg/day by continuous infusion.
  - 12–17 years: starting dose by intravenous injection 10 mg/kg, increasing up to 2.5 g/day in 2–4 divided doses by intravenous infusion or injection or up to 2.5 g/day by continuous infusion; maintenance dose 1–2 g/day (or 20–30 mg/kg/day) with intravenous injection administered over 3–5 minutes.
  - Switching from oral to intravenous therapy: give the same dose as current oral daily dose over 3–5 minutes by injection or in 2–4 divided doses by infusion.

Contraindications. Acute porphyrias, known or suspected mitochondrial disorders, personal or family history of severe hepatic dysfunction, and urea cycle disorders.

Sodium valproate should be avoided in females approaching or of childbearing age unless no other ASM has been effective in controlling seizures, because of 10% birth defects and 30–40% risk of developmental delay in pregnancy (see Chapter 8). In the UK, regulations governing the use of sodium valproate in males of reproductive age have also recently been strengthened (see Chapter 8).

Most common side effects. Dose-related tremor, weight gain due to appetite stimulation, abdominal pain, thinning or loss of hair (usually temporary), and menstrual irregularities including amenorrhea. Some young women develop polycystic ovary syndrome associated with obesity and hirsutism.

Significant interactions. Sodium valproate inhibits a range of hepatic metabolic processes, including oxidation, conjugation, and epoxidation reactions, particularly in phenytoin, phenobarbital, the active epoxide metabolite of carbamazepine, and lamotrigine. Dual therapy with sodium valproate and lamotrigine is effective but dose adjustment of lamotrigine is recommended to prevent toxicity. Sodium valproate can also increase exposure to rufinamide. Combined treatment with cannabidiol increases alanine transaminase (ALT) concentrations, necessitating 6-monthly ALT monitoring and dose adjustment as required.

There is a risk of hepatoxicity with sodium valproate and other drugs, such as statins (atorvastatin, simvastatin), antibiotics (doxycycline, flucloxacillin, oxytetracycline), immunosuppressants (methotrexate), and analgesics (paracetamol [acetaminophen]). Sodium valproate should be withdrawn immediately if the patient has hepatic dysfunction with persistent vomiting, abdominal pain, weight loss, jaundice, or deterioration in seizure control. Equally, if a patient develops pancreatitis.

Tips to aid adherence. Slower introduction in divided doses can be beneficial, especially when adding sodium valproate to lamotrigine. Patients who often forget morning or evening medication when the drug is given in divided doses can take one dose at night. The normal half-life is around 8–12 hours, although this may be up to 50% less in children aged 2–10 years (or significantly longer in infants or neonates), which would theoretically preclude this. Modified-release tablets or granules prolong the half-life slightly and are generally preferred as they tend to be better tolerated than enteric-coated preparations.

Other considerations. Liver function should be monitored before therapy and within the first 6 months of treatment.

Stiripentol
Indications. Adjunctive treatment in combination with sodium valproate and clobazam for drug-resistant GTCS and severe myoclonic epilepsy in infancy (DS).

Mechanism of action. Enhances central GABAergic neurotransmission by increasing GABA release, thereby prolonging the inhibitory effect of GABA.

Dose and administration. By mouth. Capsules (250 mg, 500 mg), powder sachets for oral suspension (250 mg, 500 mg). Stiripentol should be administered under expert supervision.

- 1 month to 5 years: starting dose 20 mg/kg/day in 2–3 divided doses for 1 week, increasing to 30 mg/kg/day in 2–3 divided doses for 1 week, then to 50 mg/kg/day in 2–3 divided doses.
- 6–11 years: starting dose 20 mg/kg/day in 2–3 divided doses for 1 week, increasing weekly by 10 mg/kg/day in 2–3 divided doses to 50 mg/kg/day in 2–3 divided doses.
- 12–17 years: starting dose: 20 mg/kg/day in 2–3 divided doses for 1 week, increasing to 30 mg/kg/day in 2–3 divided doses for 1 week, then by 5 mg/kg/day in 2–3 divided doses every week until the optimum dose is reached based on clinical judgment; maximum dose 50 mg/kg/day.

Contraindications. History of psychosis.

Most common side effects. Drowsiness, slowing of cognitive function, ataxia, diplopia, anorexia, weight loss, nausea, abdominal pain, and asymptomatic neutropenia.

Significant interactions. Stiripentol increases the concentration of carbamazepine, clobazam, phenobarbital, phenytoin, fenfluramine, and primidone; careful monitoring and potential dose adjustment are therefore required. It is also predicted to increase the concentration of aminophylline and theophylline.

Other considerations. A full blood count and liver function tests should be performed before initiating treatment and every 6 months thereafter, and growth should be monitored. The manufacturer advises avoidance of milk, dairy products, carbonated drinks, fruit juices, or caffeine-containing food and drinks when taking the medication. Capsules and oral powder are not bioequivalent; therefore, switching should be monitored because of the risk of toxicity.

Tiagabine

Indications. Adjunctive treatment for focal-onset seizures with or without bilateral tonic-clonic seizures that are not satisfactorily controlled by other ASM.

Mechanism of action. Selectively inhibits the neuronal and glial reuptake of GABA, thereby enhancing GABA-mediated inhibition.

Dose and administration. By mouth. Tablets (5 mg, 10 mg, 15 mg), oral suspension (special order).

- 12–17 years: starting dose 5–10 mg/day in 1–2 divided doses, increasing weekly by 5–10 mg/day; maintenance dose 30–45 mg/ day in 2–3 divided doses if given in combination with enzyme-inducing ASM or 15–30 mg/day in 2–3 divided doses if given with non-enzyme-inducing ASM.

Contraindications. Acute porphyrias.

Most common side effects. Dizziness, asthenia, nervousness, tremor, impaired concentration, lethargy, and depression. Weakness due to transient loss of tone can occur at high doses. The most common reasons for discontinuation of therapy are confusion, somnolence, ataxia, and dizziness. An acute psychotic reaction can develop, particularly in patients with a previous history of psychiatric disease.

Significant interactions. Carbamazepine, phenytoin, and phenobarbital decrease exposure to tiagabine, thereby lowering its plasma concentrations. St John's wort is contraindicated as it significantly reduces levels of tiagabine, leading to a loss of efficacy.

Tips to aid adherence. Patients should be advised to take tiagabine with or just after food to avoid rapid rises in plasma concentration.

Other considerations. Tiagabine may worsen absence, myoclonic, tonic, and atonic seizures.

Topiramate

Indications. Monotherapy and adjunctive treatment for focal-onset seizures with or without bilateral tonic-clonic seizures and GTCS. Also, adjunctive treatment for seizures associated with LGS.

Mechanism of action. Topiramate is a sulfamate-substituted monosaccharide that has multiple pharmacological actions involving blockade of sodium channels and high-voltage-activated calcium channels, attenuation of kainate-induced responses, and enhancement of GABAergic neurotransmission. It also inhibits carbonic anhydrase, an effect that contributes to its side-effect profile.

Dose and administration. Tablets (25 mg, 50 mg, 100 mg, 200 mg), capsules (15 mg, 25 mg, 50 mg), oral suspension (50 mg/5 mL, 100 mg/5 mL).

- Monotherapy (6–17 years): starting dose 0.5–1 mg/kg at night (maximum per dose 25 mg) for 1 week, increasing by 250–500 µg/kg bd every 1–2 weeks (maximum increase 25 mg bd); maintenance dose 50 mg bd (maximum per dose 7.5 mg/kg bd); maximum dose 500 mg/day.
- Adjunctive treatment (2–17 years): starting dose 1–3 mg/kg at night (maximum per dose 25 mg) for 1 week, increasing by 0.5–1.5 mg/ kg bd every 1–2 weeks (maximum increase 25 mg bd); maintenance dose 2.5–4.5 mg/kg bd (maximum per dose 7.5 mg/kg bd); maximum dose 400 mg/day.

Contraindications. Acute porphyrias and history of kidney stones (risk of metabolic acidosis and nephrolithiasis). Patients may experience severe abdominal pain, constipation, behavioral change, and high blood pressure.

Most common side effects. Ataxia, poor concentration, confusion, dysphasia, dizziness, fatigue, paresthesia, somnolence, word-finding difficulties, cognitive slowing, anorexia, and poor appetite/weight loss. An acute psychotic reaction can develop, particularly in patients with a previous history of psychiatric disease.

Significant interactions. Topiramate increases the risk of carbamazepine and sodium valproate toxicity when these drugs are administered concurrently. Carbamazepine, phenobarbital, and phenytoin decrease the concentration of topiramate and topiramate increases the concentration of phenytoin. At doses over 200 mg/day, topiramate decreases the efficacy of estrogen and can lead to contraceptive failure for girls taking an OCP. Topiramate potentially increases the risk of overheating and dehydration when given with zonisamide, so this concurrent use should be avoided.

Tips to aid adherence. If the child or young person cannot tolerate the recommended titration regimens described above, then smaller increases in dose or longer intervals between dose increases may be used. The risk of neurocognitive side effects can be minimized by titrating the dose slowly. The content of the capsule can be sprinkled on soft food and swallowed without chewing.

Other considerations. Overheating should be avoided and patients educated to ensure adequate hydration, especially children, and during strenuous activity or if in a warm environment.

Vigabatrin

Indications. Adjunctive treatment for focal-onset seizures with or without bilateral tonic-clonic seizures not satisfactorily controlled with other ASM. Also, monotherapy (or with prednisolone) for infantile spasms.

Mechanism of action. Inhibition of GABA transaminase, the enzyme responsible for the metabolic degradation of GABA.

Dose and administration. By mouth or by rectum. Tablets (500 mg), soluble tablets (100 mg, 500 mg), powder sachets (500 mg). Vigabatrin should be administered under expert supervision.

- Adjunctive treatment (by mouth or by rectum)
  - Neonate to 23 months: oral (or rectal in children ≥1 month) starting dose 15–20 mg/kg bd (maximum per dose 250 mg in children 1–23 months), increasing over 2–3 weeks to maintenance dose 30–40 mg/kg bd (maximum per dose 75 mg/kg).
  - 2–11 years: starting dose 15–20 mg/kg bd (maximum per dose 250 mg), increasing over 2–3 weeks to maintenance dose 30–40 mg/kg bd (maximum per dose 1.5 g).
  - 12–17 years: starting dose 250 mg bd, increasing over 2–3 weeks to maintenance dose 1–1.5 g bd.
- Monotherapy (or with prednisolone) for infantile spasms
  - 1–23 months: starting dose 25 mg/kg bd on day 1, followed by 50 mg/kg bd on days 2–4, increasing according to response up to maximum dose 75 mg/kg bd from day 5 if spasms continue.

Contraindications. Visual field defects affect up to 40% of patients. Onset of visual impairment varies from 1 month to a few years and visual field defects may persist and worsen despite discontinuation of vigabatrin. Visual field testing should be conducted before starting treatment and then at 6-monthly intervals.

Most common side effects. Tiredness, dizziness, headache, and increased appetite/weight gain. Some patients report a change in mood, commonly agitation, ill temper, disturbed behavior, or depression. An acute psychotic reaction can develop, particularly in patients with a previous history of psychiatric disease.

Significant interactions. Vigabatrin reduces the concentration of phenytoin.

Tips to aid adherence. Granular powder formulations should be dissolved in water, fruit juice, or milk immediately before they are taken.

Other considerations. The dose should be reduced, or the dose interval increased, if creatinine clearance is less than 60 mL/minute. Close monitoring of neurological function is recommended. It should be noted that vigabatrin can worsen absences and myoclonic jerks.

Zonisamide

Indications. Adjunctive treatment for drug-resistant focal seizures with or without bilateral tonic-clonic seizures.

Off-label use. Monotherapy for focal-onset seizures with or without bilateral tonic-clonic seizures in newly diagnosed epilepsy. Monotherapy and adjunctive treatment for GTCS.

Mechanism of action. Blocks voltage-dependent sodium and T-type calcium channels, and actively inhibits the release of excitatory neurotransmitters.

Dose and administration. By mouth. Capsules (25 mg, 50 mg, 100 mg), oral suspension (20 mg/mL), oral suspension/solution 10 mg/mL (special order).

- 6–17 years (bodyweight 20–54 kg): starting dose 1 mg/kg/day for 7 days, increasing by 1 mg/kg every 7 days to maintenance dose 6–8 mg/kg/day (maximum per dose 500 mg/day); dose to be increased every 2 weeks in patients who are not receiving concomitant carbamazepine, phenytoin, phenobarbital, or other potent inducers of cytochrome P450 enzyme CYP3A4.
- 6–17 years (bodyweight ≥55 kg): starting dose 1 mg/kg/day for 7 days, increasing by 1 mg/kg every 7 days to maintenance dose 300–500 mg/day; dose to be increased every 2 weeks in patients who are not receiving concomitant carbamazepine, phenytoin, phenobarbital, or other potent inducers of cytochrome P450 enzyme CYP3A4.

Contraindications. Theoretical hypersensitivity syndrome, such as risk of rash.

Most common side effects. Anxiety, mood changes, decreased appetite, weight loss, cognitive impairment, somnolence, gastrointestinal discomfort, dizziness, ataxia, and fatigue.

Significant interactions. Phenytoin, carbamazepine, and phenobarbital decrease the half-life of zonisamide by approximately 50%. Lamotrigine increases zonisamide concentrations. Zonisamide can reduce the carbamazepine-10,11-epoxide to carbamazepine ratio. Zonisamide should be avoided in children treated concomitantly with carbonic anhydrase inhibitors such as topiramate and acetazolamide, because of the potential risk of overheating and dehydration.

Tips to aid adherence. A slower titration rate can be applied if necessary. Zonisamide's relatively long half-life (49–69 hours in monotherapy) means that once-daily administration is possible, particularly when a stable dose has been reached.

Other considerations. Patients with renal dysfunction have lower rates of clearance, so zonisamide should be discontinued if renal function deteriorates. Caution is advised in patients with risk factors for renal stone formation (particularly a predisposition for nephrolithiasis). Overheating should be avoided and patients educated to ensure adequate hydration, especially children, or during strenuous activity or if in a warm environment. Fatal cases of heat stroke have been reported in children.

Monitor serum bicarbonate concentration in children and those with other risk factors such as renal disease, severe respiratory disorders, or diarrhea; dose reduction or discontinuation should be considered if metabolic acidosis develops.

Weight should be monitored throughout treatment, as fatal cases of weight loss have been reported in children.

Key points – pharmacological treatment

- ASM should be prescribed for CYPWE when they have experienced two or more seizures.
- ASM prevent seizures by decreasing excitation or enhancing inhibition of neurons.
- Verbal and written information should be provided about the risk of seizure recurrence, the likelihood of remission of seizures, the likely duration of treatment, and the risks and benefits of treatment. The importance of adherence to prescribed medication should also be emphasized.
- The choice of ASM depends on the type of seizures, concomitant medication, and underlying health conditions, as well as the potential longevity of the epilepsy.
- ASM should be started at low doses and titrated slowly. Serum ASM levels should then be monitored to assess the effectiveness of treatment and to prevent or minimize side effects.
- ASM should be increased within the limits of tolerability, with the goal of achieving complete seizure freedom.

References

1. Bromfield EB, Cavazos JE, Sirven JI, eds. Neuropharmacology of antiepileptic drugs. In: *An Introduction to Epilepsy [Internet].* American Epilepsy Society, 2006.

2. Martin M, Hill C, Bewley S et al. Transgenerational adverse effects of valproate? A patient report from 90 affected families. *Birth Defects Res* 2022;114:13–16.

3. National Institute for Health and Care Excellence (NICE). *Epilepsies in children, young people and adults. NICE guideline [NG217].* NICE, 2022. nice.org.uk/guidance/ng217, last accessed 1 November 2023.

4. National Institute for Health and Care Excellence (NICE). *British National Formulary for Children (BNFC).* NICE, 2023. bnfc.nice.org.uk, last accessed 1 November 2023.

5. Electronic Medicines Compendium (emc). *Summary of Product Characteristics (SmPC): Ontozry.* medicines.org.uk/emc/company/4195, last accessed 1 November 2023.

6. Varughese RT, Shah YD, Karkare S, Kothare SV. Adjunctive use of cenobamate for pediatric refractory focal-onset epilepsy: a single-center retrospective study. *Epilepsy Behav* 2022;130:108679.

7. Makridis KL, Bast T, Prager C et al. Real-world experience treating epilepsy patients with cenobamate. *Front Neurol* 2022;13:950171.

8. Smith MC, Klein P, Krauss GL et al. Dose adjustment of concomitant antiseizure medications during cenobamate treatment: expert opinion consensus recommendations. *Neurol Ther* 2022;11:1705–20.

9. Osborn M, Abou-Khalil B. The cenobamate-clobazam interaction – evidence of synergy in addition to pharmacokinetic interaction. *Epilepsy Behav* 2023;142:109156.

6 Non-pharmacological management

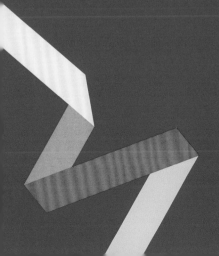

HEALTHCARE

Ketogenic diet

The ketogenic diet (KD) is a specialized treatment initiated in tertiary care for drug-resistant or refractory epilepsy. The traditional KD is a high fat, very low carbohydrate diet, with adequate protein for growth. It causes metabolic changes in the body, such that fat is burned for energy instead of glucose, producing more ketone bodies, a state known as ketosis (see Mechanism of action, below). Different ratios of fat to protein plus carbohydrate can be prescribed (4:1, 3:1, 2:1); the most common is the 3:1 ratio (3 g of fat to 1 g of protein and carbohydrate combined).

The KD should be considered for children and young people with epilepsy (CYPWE) who have:
- a childhood-onset epilepsy syndrome
- glucose transporter 1 deficiency syndrome (Glut1DS)
- pyruvate dehydrogenase deficiency
- infantile spasms
- epilepsy with myoclonic-atonic seizures
- Dravet syndrome (DS)
- Lennox–Gastaut syndrome (LGS)
- drug-resistant epilepsy.

Mechanism of action. The exact mechanism by which the KD exerts its antiseizure effect is unknown. The KD appears to mimic starvation by using free fatty acids as an alternative fuel source for the body. These are converted into ketone bodies, which are thought to reduce the excitability of neurons, thereby reducing the tendency for seizures. There is also anecdotal evidence to suggest that motor coordination, cognition, and behavior improve, alongside an improvement in the level of alertness, in CYPWE who adopt a KD.[1]

Diet variations. Compared with the traditional KD described above, the medium chain triglyceride (MCT) KD allows more carbohydrate and protein because some of the fat is substituted with a source of MCT (an oil or emulsion). The MCT increases ketosis, so the overall fat content of the diet can be reduced.

Two modified versions of the KD have also been developed. The modified Atkins diet is a low carbohydrate, high fat diet that does not limit or measure protein or total calories. The low glycemic index diet allows more carbohydrate, but it is only suitable for individuals with a glycemic index lower than 50. Both modified diets require nutritional supplementation. More detailed information about the different KD therapies can be found at matthewsfriends.org.

Managing the effects of a ketogenic diet. Most CYPWE remain on the KD for about 2 years. Those who cannot tolerate the diet, or whose seizures worsen while on it, will discontinue sooner. Children with Glut1DS often continue the KD into adulthood, with the support of medical professionals with expertise in managing the diet.

Parents and caregivers of CYPWE taking the KD should be counseled on its side effects (Table 6.1) and the regular monitoring that is required.[2] This should include discussion of dietary restrictions, blood monitoring during the initiation phase, regular ongoing monitoring, and recognizing and responding to abnormal glucose levels when CYPWE are unwell. Support for parents and caregivers can include handouts, training videos, and support groups, in addition to regular contact with the specialist team. Training and monitoring will also be required for education and social care settings.

TABLE 6.1

Side effects of the ketogenic diet

Gastrointestinal symptoms

- Nausea and vomiting
- Diarrhea
- Abdominal pain
- Exacerbation of gastroesophageal reflux
- Constipation
- Lethargy
- Dehydration
- Weight loss

CONTINUED

TABLE 6.1 CONTINUED

Side effects of the ketogenic diet

Metabolic symptoms

- Hypercholesterolemia
- High levels of LDL cholesterol
- Elevated total cholesterol
- Hypoglycemia
- Metabolic acidosis

Renal problems

- Renal calculi (3–7% of children)

Growth and skeletal problems

- Cessation of growth
- Osteoporosis and reduced vitamin D levels (especially with concomitant ASM)

ASM, antiseizure medication; LDL, low density lipoprotein.

Monitoring. Numerous baseline blood investigations are required before starting the diet, including cholesterol, vitamin D, kidney function, liver function, acetylcholine, and serum electrolytes. An ultrasound scan of the kidneys can also be beneficial. Monitoring should be undertaken at 3 and 6 months after treatment starts and every 6 months thereafter.[2]

Vagus nerve stimulation

Vagus nerve stimulation is a palliative treatment option for patients with drug-refractory epilepsy who are not eligible for other types of surgery (see below), or for whom surgery has failed to produce adequate benefits. VNS can be used in children of all ages, regardless of epilepsy syndrome and seizure type,[3] provided the child meets the criteria for implantation set by the manufacturer and the multidisciplinary team has decided that conventional medication will have no further effectiveness. Newer, smaller VNS devices are available, which allow implantation in young children. Responder rates are lower in CYPWE with intellectual disability (ID), but this may be because of the higher prevalence of difficult-to-treat seizures in this population.[3]

Mechanism of action. The mechanism by which VNS exerts its antiseizure properties is multifactorial (Figure 6.1).[4] Action potentials generated at a cathode (negative electrode) travel afferently along the vagus nerve to the brainstem. Efferent action potentials traveling to the heart, lungs, and other organs in the body are mainly blocked by a positive electrode, thereby reducing potential side effects. Most vagal afferent synapses end in the nucleus tractus solitarius (NTS) of the brainstem. Stimulation of the NTS has been shown to increase γ-aminobutyric acid (GABA) signaling or decrease glutamate signaling.

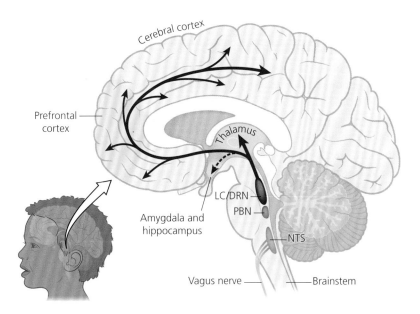

Figure 6.1 Pathways involved in vagus nerve stimulation. Action potentials travel afferently to the nucleus tractus solitarius (NTS) and subsequently project to other areas of the brainstem, including the locus ceruleus (LC), dorsal raphe nuclei (DRN), and parabrachial nucleus (PBN). Signals project from the LC to the limbic system (amygdala and hippocampus) and prefrontal cortex, from the DRN to upper areas of the cerebral cortex, and from the PBN to the thalamus.

The NTS also has projections to several key structures in the brainstem, including the locus ceruleus (LC), the dorsal raphe nuclei (DRN), and the parabrachial nucleus (PBN). VNS increases resting state autonomous firing of the LC and DRN. Stimulation of the LC suppresses epileptic activity within the amygdala. The LC and DRN are the main noradrenaline (norepinephrine) and serotonin production sites in the brain, respectively, and stimulation of these areas may account for the antidepressant effects of VNS. The NTS also has direct connections to the limbic system via the amygdala and thalamus.

VNS has been shown to prevent the lowering of seizure thresholds of neurons in the amygdala as well as potentially decreasing excitability and thereby seizure generation in the hippocampus. There are reciprocal connections between the prefrontal cortex and the brainstem, thalamus, basal ganglia, and limbic system.

Therapeutic responses to VNS are associated with the normalization of GABA-A receptor density in cortical regions. VNS has an antiseizure effect, by containing seizure propagation using a train of stimulations (described above). However, it also seems to have an anti-epileptogenic effect, given that seizures following VNS treatment are more localized or lateralized to a smaller portion of the brain and therefore may have a less severe clinical semiology.[4]

The VNS system consists of a programmable signal generator implanted in the patient's left upper chest (Figure 6.2). Bipolar leads connect the generator to the left vagus nerve in the neck. Stimulation is configured using a programming wand, which non-invasively communicates with the signal generator. A handheld magnet can be used by the patient or caregiver to provide additional stimulation when seizure triggers occur or at the onset of a seizure to limit its severity.

Newer devices, such as the SenTiva and Aspire SR, incorporate autostimulation based on changes in heart rate, which occur at seizure onset, with the aim of aborting it. As 82% of CYPWE experience ictal tachycardia, this use of heart rate detection has proven an effective method of improving the efficacy of the device.[5] Heart rate detection is recorded to provide a baseline, and the parameters for VNS activation are set at 20–40% above this. Low heart rates can

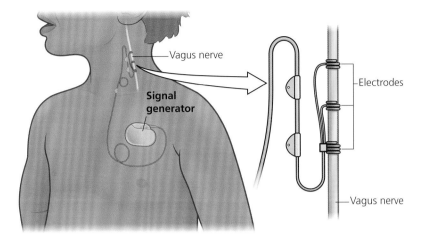

Figure 6.2 Vagus nerve stimulation system. A signal generator is implanted in the left upper chest wall. It is connected by a single lead to three coils that wrap around the left vagus nerve in the cervical region.

also be detected. Consideration needs to be given to non-seizure-related or exercise-induced changes in heart rate, which may trigger a stimulation.[5]

Before implantation children/parents and caregivers should be counseled to understand:

- the risks of surgery
- the importance of monitoring for side effects
- the importance of regular follow-up
- the dosing regimen
- reduction of seizure frequency and duration, potential seizure cluster reduction, and improvement in quality of life
- potential reduction of antiseizure medication (ASM) if better seizure control is achieved
- potential of further surgery for lead or battery replacement.[5]

Adverse events. Serious adverse events are rare and mainly relate to surgery. They include infection, nerve paralysis, facial paresis, and left vocal cord paralysis. Voice alteration (hoarseness) and coughing are

TABLE 6.2

Side effects of vagal nerve stimulation

Common	Uncommon
• Hoarseness	• Dyspepsia
• Voice alteration	• Vomiting
• Paresthesia	• Obstructive sleep apnea
• Cough	
• Shortness of breath	

the most common non-serious adverse events (Table 6.2), affecting approximately half of patients in clinical trials, with a wide range of severity.[6] In practice, the device is generally very well tolerated and CYPWE become accustomed to the stimulation. The handheld magnet can be strapped across the device to temporarily turn off stimulation, for example if the child has a sore throat.

Stimulation titration. The VNS device is generally turned on a couple of weeks after implantation. Stimulation is then titrated, in terms of signal frequency and 'on-time' versus 'off time', according to clinical effect and tolerability. Optimal effects are usually only seen many months, or even a couple of years, after implantation.

VNS is dosed in milliamps (mA) of electrical current and, like ASM, it is titrated on a regular basis after implantation. Newer devices have a programmable feature to autotitrate stimulation to a level that is tolerated by the individual. Once this tolerable level is reached, the strength of stimulus (output current) and pulse width (number of pulses per second) can be set. The magnet mode of output current is always set at 0.25 mA above the normal current to prepare the child or young person for the next automatic titration to ensure they tolerate the higher dose.[6]

Therapy is delivered at set intervals throughout the day, varying between 10% and 58% of a day (duty cycle), and the time between on/off can vary according to the individual's tolerance or seizure type. Close collaboration between the manufacturer representative and the clinician will optimize the potential of the device.[6]

As mentioned above, the newer SenTiva device also has an autostimulation or 'AutoStim' feature, which automatically generates an impulse when it detects an increase in heart rate.[6] Additional features of VNS include:

- day/night programming
- an events tab to review hourly and daily trends in normal, auto, and magnet stimulations
- detection of low/high heart rate.

Surgery

Indications. Surgery should be considered as an option in CYPWE who have drug-resistant or refractory epilepsy, with the aim of reducing seizure burden and the risk of cognitive decline and mortality associated with medically refractory epilepsy. The approach to epilepsy surgery in CYPWE is different from adults for several reasons (Table 6.3).[7]

Referral. International best practice recommends that CYPWE are referred to tertiary neurology services if there is diagnostic uncertainty, and if specialized advice on drugs and surgery is required. Indications for referral are shown in Table 6.4.[8]

TABLE 6.3

Reasons for epilepsy surgery in children and young people

- Seizure frequency is much higher in CYPWE than adults
- Frequent and recurrent seizures in CYPWE increase the incidence of developmental arrest or regression, especially in children under 2 years old
- Focal seizures in CYPWE are often associated with age-specific causes; focal cortical dysplasias, which are often caused by prolonged convulsive seizures, are more common in children
- Localization-related epilepsy is often diverse in CYPWE where there is a rapid onset of seizures with electroclinical features
- Thorough early surgical planning is required to preserve neuroplasticity and functional reorganization of nerve pathways within the developing brain

CYPWE, children and young people with epilepsy.

TABLE 6.4

Indications for referral to a tertiary epilepsy center

- The epilepsy is not controlled with medication within 2 years of onset
- Management is unsuccessful after two drugs
- The child is under 2 years old
- The child or young person experiences, or is at risk of, unacceptable side effects from medication
- Unilateral structural lesion
- Psychological or psychiatric comorbidity
- Diagnostic doubt as to the nature of the seizures or the seizure syndrome

Presurgical assessment. A specialized multidisciplinary service assesses CYPWE who are eligible for epilepsy surgery on an individual basis following referral to their tertiary center. The presurgical assessment involves an extensive series of investigations to identify if the child or young person is suitable for surgery (Table 6.5).[8]

Types of surgery. Once the assessment is completed, both the referring center and the parents/caregivers will be informed if surgery is an option. The type of surgery offered will depend on the types of seizures and where they occur in the brain.[8]

The primary goal of surgery is to address the epileptogenic area, which is not always where the lesion is.[9] For this reason, there must be correlation between radiographic and epileptogenic localization.

There are two types of epilepsy surgery:

- resective operations, such as lesionectomy and temporal lobectomy
- disconnective procedures, such as corpus callosotomy and hemispherectomy.[10]

Lesionectomy is surgical resection of the lesion causing the seizures. These may be focal cortical dysplasias, low-grade tumors, or cavernous arterial and arteriovenous malformations. Outcomes

TABLE 6.5

Presurgical investigations

* EEG/video telemetry
* Invasive EEG telemetry
* MRI
* Functional MRI
* PET scan
* SPECT scan
* MEG scan
* Neuropsychology tests
* Neuropsychiatry tests
* Other assessments

EEG, electroencephalography; MEG, magnetoencephalography; MRI, magnetic resonance imaging; PET, positron emission tomography; SPECT, single-photon emission computed tomography.

following surgery are variable. The extent of the lesionectomy has been shown to correlate with seizure freedom. Postoperative complications such as infections, hemiparesis, dysphasia, and visual field defects are very low.[10]

Temporal lobectomy is surgical resection of the anterior temporal lobe. This has been shown to be the most effective technique used in practice as there may be dual pathology involving both the amygdala and the hippocampus.[9] Temporal lobectomy often has a favorable outcome, and case series show complete seizure freedom (Engel class I; Table 6.6) in over 70% of cases.[10]

Corpus callosotomy is a palliative option that aims to reduce seizure burden and the negative effects that frequent seizures bring. Corpus callosotomy involves transecting most or all of the corpus callosum to disconnect communication between the two hemispheres. Case series have demonstrated a significant reduction in atonic and tonic seizures in CYPWE who have this procedure. Complete seizure freedom rates (Engel class I) are lower in this group at 10–20%.[10,11]

TABLE 6.6

ILAE surgical outcome (Engel) classification scales[11]

Classification	Outcome
Class I	Seizure free
Class II	Auras only
Class III	1–3 seizure days per year, and auras
Class IV	4 seizure days per year to 50% reduction in baseline, and auras
Class V	<50% reduction in baseline number of seizure days to 100% increase in baseline number of seizure days and auras
Class VI	>100% increase in baseline number of seizure days and auras

ILAE, International League Against Epilepsy.

Hemispherectomy is a resection of half of the child's brain; it is either totally or partially removed or disconnected from the rest of the brain. Following surgery, two-thirds of children become completely seizure free and a further 15–20% experience a substantial reduction in seizures.[12] CYPWE often have hemiplegia both pre- and postoperatively.[10]

Practical considerations. Before surgery, CYPWE and their families will need to be counseled on the benefits, risks, and potential complications of the surgery. As the surgery is performed in highly specialized centers that may not be local to the child's home, parents will need support to ensure they can attend all presurgical appointments and have adequate financial, family, and social support both during and after surgery.

Education settings will also need to be aware of the potential time for recovery after surgery. Neurocognitive evaluation before surgery will help to identify cognitive strengths and difficulties so that areas of potential support can be recommended.

Risks. The risks of epilepsy surgery depend on the type of surgery. They include infection, bleeding, brain swelling, problems with memory, partial loss of sight, and dense hemiplegia, which may or may not recover over time. Mortality is low at 0.5–1%.[9]

Recovery. Postoperative recovery may involve specialist neurological intensive care for the first 24–48 hours, again depending on the type of surgery. Most CYPWE will have an inpatient stay of 3–4 days, and full recovery from surgery may take about 3–4 weeks. There can be an initial decline in cognition and memory, which often resolves within a year of surgery.[12]

Key points – non-pharmacological management

- Non-pharmacological approaches to treatment should be considered when the child or young person has failed to achieve adequate seizure control with two ASM.
- Alternative non-pharmacological interventions must be decided via a multidisciplinary team approach, taking into account the individual needs of CYPWE and their families.
- The KD is a high fat, low carbohydrate regimen initiated in tertiary care for drug-resistant or refractory epilepsy. Regular monitoring is required.
- VNS is the treatment of choice for children with drug-refractory epilepsy who are not eligible for other types of surgery, or for whom surgery has failed to produce adequate benefits. VNS can be used in children of all ages, regardless of epilepsy syndrome and seizure type. Serious adverse events are rare.
- Various types of epilepsy surgery are available. Surgery addresses the epileptogenic area, which is not always where the lesion is. Correlation between radiographic and epileptogenic localization is therefore essential.
- Discussion of VNS and surgical options for epilepsy should include the potential benefits, complications, and risks.

References

1. Hallböök T, Ji S, Maudsley S, Martin B. The effects of the ketogenic diet on behavior and cognition. *Epilepsy Res* 2012;100:304–9.
2. National Institute for Health and Care Excellence. *Epilepsies in children, young people and adults: diagnosis and management. [12] Evidence review: ketogenic diets for drug-resistant epilepsy. NICE guideline [NG217].* NICE, 2022. nice.org.uk/guidance/ng217/documents/evidence-review-19, last accessed 1 November 2023.
3. Sourbron J, Klinkenberg S, Kessels A et al. Vagus nerve stimulation in children: a focus on intellectual disability. *Eur J Paediatr Neurol* 2017;21:427–40.
4. Carron R, Roncon P, Lagarde S et al. Latest views on the mechanisms of action of surgically implanted cervical vagal nerve stimulation in epilepsy. *Neuromodulation* 2023;26:498–506.
5. Fisher B, DesMarteau JA, Koontz EH et al. Responsive vagus nerve stimulation for drug resistant epilepsy: a review of new features and practical guidance for advanced practice providers. *Front Neurol* 2020;11:610379.
6. LivaNova Epilepsy. *VNS Therapy® System Epilepsy Physician's Manual (EU).* LivaNova, 2020. livanova.com/epilepsy-vnstherapy/en-gb/hcp/physician-manuals, last accessed 1 November 2023.
7. Jayalakshmi S, Vooturi S, Gupta S, Panigrahi M. Epilepsy surgery in children. *Neurol India* 2017;65:485–92.
8. Epilepsy Action. *Children's Epilepsy Surgery Service in England (CESS).* Epilepsy Action, 2021 (modified 2023). epilepsy.org.uk/info/treatment/surgery/children, last accessed 1 November 2023.
9. Braun KPJ, Cross JH. Pediatric epilepsy surgery: the earlier the better. *Expert Rev Neurother* 2018;18:261–3.
10. Dallas J, Englot DJ, Naftel RP. Neurosurgical approaches to pediatric epilepsy: indications, techniques, and outcomes of common surgical procedures. *Seizure* 2020;77:76–85.
11. Weiser HG, Blume WT, Fish D et al. ILAE commission report. Proposal for a new classification of outcome with respect to epileptic seizures following epilepsy surgery. *Epilepsia* 2001;42:282–6.
12. Chugani HT, Asano E, Juhász C et al. "Subtotal" hemispherectomy in children with intractable focal epilepsy. *Epilepsia* 2014;55:1926–33.

7 Comorbidities and complications

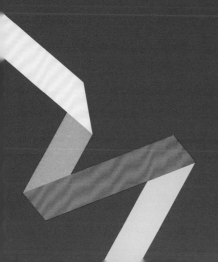

Comorbidities are more common in children and young people with epilepsy (CYPWE) than in the general population. They include psychiatric, neurological, and cognitive conditions and can occur either singularly or in combination. It is important to identify comorbid conditions from the time of diagnosis as they will affect treatment options, response to treatment, medical costs, and quality of life.[1–3] A few studies have identified a bidirectional relationship between epilepsy and comorbid psychiatric and cognitive conditions.[3,4]

Mental health issues

The incidence of psychiatric disorders has been reported to be significantly higher in children with epilepsy (37%) than peers with diabetes (11%) or in a control group (9%).[1] Multiple facets of the epilepsies may affect the mental health of children and young people, including the frequency, type or severity of seizures, cognitive impairment, structural brain abnormalities, behavioral or emotional side effects of antiseizure medication (ASM), and family/psychosocial factors.[2] There is a bidirectional relationship between anxiety/depression and epilepsy: anxiety and depression can increase seizure frequency, and seizures can worsen anxiety and depression.[3]

Anxiety markedly compromises quality of life and psychosocial functioning. Ictal anxiety may be mistaken for a panic disorder. The severity of anxiety does not necessarily correlate with seizure frequency. In the CHESS study, separation and physical injury were reported by both children and parents as causes of anxiety.[4] However, parents and children may identify different anxieties, so it is important to determine the views of CYPWE, taking into consideration their age, understanding, and any intellectual disability (ID). Older children have been found to identify more symptoms of anxiety than younger children.

Depression. A 2011 systematic review of evidence from population-based studies suggested that the prevalence of depression in children with epilepsy is 12–14%.[5] However, depression in the general population is under-recognized and, when diagnosed, often undertreated, especially in children and young people. Diagnosis may be further complicated if the patient minimizes or internalizes their symptoms, or if the clinician does not inquire about psychiatric symptoms or considers depression to be part of the normal adaptation to the diagnosis of epilepsy. A significantly high rate of self-injurious behavior and suicidal ideation has been identified in CYPWE, increasing the risk of suicide attempts.[6] Thus, the consequence of underdiagnosis and undertreatment can be fatal.

Seizure type, especially generalized tonic-clonic seizures (GTCS), can have a significant effect on depression scores. This may be due to the loss of consciousness and visibility of this type of seizure.[4] GTCS are also more likely to be associated with working memory deficits, which may affect school and home life, potentially exacerbating symptoms of anxiety or depression.[5]

Assessment. There are many simple screening instruments that can rapidly detect symptoms of anxiety and depression in busy clinical settings, but they may not be age or epilepsy specific. While no screening tool is perfect, the NDDI-E-Y (Neurological Disorders Depression Inventory-Epilepsy for Youth) is a self-report means of assessing depressive symptoms that has been validated for use in young people aged 12–17 years with a sensitivity of 79% and a specificity of 92% (Figure 7.1).[7] This tool can easily be used for initial and follow-up screening in a busy clinic. Screening should be repeated every 6 months, when there is a worsening of seizures, after changes to medication, or if any concerns are raised by the parents or caregivers regarding the child or young person's mood or behavior.

Management. It is not sufficient to purely identify symptoms of anxiety and depression; there must be clear pathways for referral for treatment with the aim of reducing the impact of anxiety or depression on the overall quality of life of CYPWE.

Many ASM have a negative psychotropic action, including topiramate, levetiracetam, zonisamide, and perampanel, as well as those with a GABAergic mode of action (see Chapter 5). These ASM can increase the risk of depression in CYPWE, especially if initiated at, or titrated rapidly to, a high dose. Conversely, some ASM, such as sodium valproate, carbamazepine, oxcarbazepine, and lamotrigine, are known to have an antidepressant or mood-stabilizing effect.[8] From the epilepsy clinician's perspective, if a patient is taking an ASM that

The NDDI-E-Y

Mark the answer that best describes how often you have had the following feelings and thoughts within the past 2 weeks.

1. Everything is a struggle
◯ Never ◯ Rarely ◯ Sometimes ◯ Very often or always

2. I have trouble finding anything that makes me happy
◯ Never ◯ Rarely ◯ Sometimes ◯ Very often or always

3. I feel like crying
◯ Never ◯ Rarely ◯ Sometimes ◯ Very often or always

4. I feel frustrated
◯ Never ◯ Rarely ◯ Sometimes ◯ Very often or always

5. I feel unhappy
◯ Never ◯ Rarely ◯ Sometimes ◯ Very often or always

6. I think about dying or killing myself
◯ Never ◯ Rarely ◯ Sometimes ◯ Very often or always

7. Nothing I do is ever right
◯ Never ◯ Rarely ◯ Sometimes ◯ Very often or always

8. I feel sorry about things
◯ Never ◯ Rarely ◯ Sometimes ◯ Very often or always

9. I feel sad
◯ Never ◯ Rarely ◯ Sometimes ◯ Very often or always

10. I feel guilty
◯ Never ◯ Rarely ◯ Sometimes ◯ Very often or always

11. I feel cranky or irritated
◯ Never ◯ Rarely ◯ Sometimes ◯ Very often or always

12. I feel alone
◯ Never ◯ Rarely ◯ Sometimes ◯ Very often or always

(Never = 0; Rarely = 1; Sometimes = 2; Very often or always = 3)
A total score of 32 is the cut-off for depression.
A high score (2 or 3) on item 6 may indicate suicidality.

Figure 7.1 The Neurological Disorders Depression Inventory-Epilepsy for Youth (NDDI-E-Y): a screening tool for depressive symptoms in pediatric epilepsy. Adapted from Wagner et al. 2016.[7]

is or may be enhancing symptoms of anxiety or depression, including suicidal ideation, consideration should be given to switching to another ASM that has a low(er) risk of worsening psychiatric symptoms.

Cognitive behavioral therapy (CBT), sertraline, or a combination of both have been shown to treat childhood anxiety disorders effectively. However, these findings are not specific to epilepsy.[9] Outcomes from studies such as the Mental Health Intervention for Children with Epilepsy (MICE) project may provide more guidance with regards to the most effective treatments in CYPWE.[10]

Non-pharmacological interventions for depression include psychoeducation around epilepsy, its treatment, and associated learning and social difficulties, as well as individual/family therapy, CBT, and support from school services.[8]

For young people with moderate-to-severe depression, pharmacological treatment, initially with selective serotonin-reuptake inhibitors (SSRIs), may well be considered but must take into account tolerability, possible side effects, and possible interactions with ASM.[8] Combinations of 'talking therapy' and antidepressants are probably more effective than either type of treatment on its own.

Behavioral issues

There is a spectrum of behavioral disorders that includes attention deficit hyperactivity disorder (ADHD), autism spectrum disorder (ASD), and developmental delays.

Attention deficit hyperactivity disorder. A review of studies found that the rates of ADHD were 2–3 times higher in CYPWE than controls.[11] The inattentive presentation of ADHD was seen more frequently than the combined presentation of attention deficit and hyperactivity. Moreover, the condition was often present at the time of, or before, the first seizure. Factors associated with a higher risk for ADHD include complicated or refractory epilepsy, higher frequency of seizures, and earlier age of onset.[11]

Although ADHD may be a comorbidity of epilepsy, it is also important to consider whether some aspects of the underlying seizure disorder or the treatments being used may be contributing to the ADHD symptoms.

Assessment. Where there is suspicion of ADHD, a referral should be made to appropriate local child/adolescent mental health services. This may be a pediatrician with training in this area or a specialist psychiatrist for children and young people. Referral is normally via the primary care provider or sometimes by the epilepsy specialist.

Management. First-line treatment for children under 5 years old usually comprises group parent-training programs and environment modification, with the addition of individual parent-training programs where the need is complex or there is difficulty attending group sessions. Medication can be considered for children over 5 years old, but only if the ADHD is causing significant persistent impairment in at least one of the following areas:

- social skills with peers
- problem-solving
- self-control
- active listening skills
- dealing with and expressing feelings.

Baseline assessment of mental and physical health, including medical history, current medications, height, weight, pulse, and blood pressure should be performed along with a baseline cardiovascular assessment.

Stimulants are the recommended first-line pharmacological treatment for ADHD: initially methylphenidate, then lisdexamfetamine, dexamfetamine, or atomoxetine, depending on age and tolerability.[12] There have been concerns that these medications may increase seizure frequency, but there is no evidence to support this. However, stimulants can cause insomnia and/or affect sleep architecture,[13] which is known to lower the seizure threshold. It is therefore sensible to ask parents and school staff to monitor seizure frequency during the initiation of these medications.[11]

A course of CBT may be considered for children over 5 years old who have benefited from medication but still have symptoms in one of the areas listed above.

Autism spectrum disorder. The link between ASD and epilepsy is not clearly understood. Individuals with epilepsy have an increased risk of ASD, especially those who are diagnosed with epilepsy in early childhood. Conversely, there is a higher incidence of epilepsy in children and young people with autism.[14] Risk factors for children with ASD developing epilepsy include female sex, ID, an underlying brain abnormality, and poor verbal skills.[15] A longitudinal study in Sweden also found that the offspring and siblings of people with epilepsy were at increased risk of ASD, further suggesting a common/shared etiology.[15]

ASD has also been associated with maternal use of sodium valproate, a highly teratogenic ASM that is associated with a 10% risk of physical abnormalities and a 30–40% risk of developmental delay (see Chapter 5).

Recognizing seizures can be challenging for caregivers, as children and young people with ASD may be unable to express unusual symptoms or sensations associated with a seizure. Sensory behaviors or stereotypies may be mistaken for seizure symptoms. Conversely, seizure symptoms may be misinterpreted as sensory issues. It is important to remember that nocturnal epileptiform changes may be seen in children with autism in whom seizures have not been identified and who have no genetic problems.[16] This highlights the need for careful and comprehensive history taking when investigating any paroxysmal episodes. Home video recordings can be very helpful to differentiate seizures from other events in this cohort of patients.

Management. It is important to have a low threshold for referring children with ASD to a pediatrician with a specialist interest in epilepsy when suspected seizures occur. Conversely, it is important to observe children with epilepsy for signs of ASD and refer them for appropriate screening if any features are present. A multidisciplinary approach may be necessary, depending on the child's individual needs. This could include speech and language therapy, physiotherapy, occupational therapy, behavioral interventions, and family counseling and support.

Aggression. It is important to distinguish between aggression that occurs as part of a seizure (most frequently as part of postictal confusion) and interictal aggression. There is very little evidence available on the specific occurrence of aggression but, in general, severity and frequency of seizures are better predictors of behavioral dysfunction than seizure syndrome or type.[17]

Research suggests that some ASM may increase behavioral side effects in CYPWE (see Table 5.2); indeed, all ASM may affect mood.

As ASM have different/multiple modes of action, it is difficult to identify why they accentuate aggressive behavior.[18] Children on ASM polytherapy have significantly higher scores for aggressive behavior.[17] It is therefore important to consider whether ASM may be precipitating aggressive behavior and to balance the need for seizure control with the effect that aggression may have on a child's and their family's quality of life.

Referral to a psychologist or psychiatrist for behavioral therapy may be indicated if the child continues to exhibit aggressive behavior.

Supportive strategies. Research into the use of supportive strategies, such as relaxation or CBT, in relation to CYPWE with behavioral issues is limited. Studies on small numbers of children/young people or children and their families with autism or ADHD have shown that mindfulness-based therapies can reduce aggression. This appears to be supported by research conducted in the general child/young person population.[19]

The International League Against Epilepsy (ILAE) supports the use of therapies such as mindfulness and CBT for comorbid behavioral difficulties in people with epilepsy, although it notes that more pediatric/adolescent-specific research is required.[20] It is also important to acknowledge that family therapy as well as individual therapy may be beneficial for the quality of life of all parties.

Intellectual disabilities

The prevalence of epilepsy in people with ID is 21.6%, with the prevalence of epilepsy rising as ID increases (10% in individuals with mild ID to 30% in those with moderate, severe, or profound ID).[21] Diagnosis relies heavily on an accurate description of events. In particular, focal-onset seizures can be mistaken for behaviors, perhaps associated with autism, and vice versa. Seizures in Rett syndrome can be particularly problematic to diagnose.

Assessment. Although some CYPWE with ID have difficulty tolerating investigations, every attempt should be made to use the full range of diagnostic tests. More time should be allowed to explain procedures and perform the studies, and use of ambulatory EEG in the home environment should be considered. The types of seizures experienced by CYPWE with ID will vary according to the syndromic diagnosis.

Management of CYPWE with ID is complex and should be undertaken by a multidisciplinary team. Some epilepsies, such as Dravet syndrome (DS) and Lennox–Gastaut syndrome (LGS), are heavily associated with changes in cognitive function (Table 7.1),[22-25] and the seizures in these syndromes can be extremely difficult to treat. There is often a temptation to use high-dose polypharmacy to manage the seizures, but this may be detrimental to overall quality of life.

Given that ASM exert their effect by enhancing inhibitory neurotransmission or suppressing neuronal excitability, it is no surprise that they may directly affect cognitive function (see Table 5.2), either by causing further cognitive impairment or in the case of a few medications providing limited cognitive benefits.[26] In general, higher doses of ASM and polypharmacy increase the risk of cognitive side effects.[26] Families should be informed about the possible cognitive side effects of ASM, and cognition should be reviewed during clinical appointments and as necessary with education providers.

Despite the challenges of pharmacological treatment in this population, pediatricians must resist any feelings of nihilism and make every effort to reduce an individual's seizure burden. Often, 'fresh eyes' can transform lives.[27] There is certainly a role for vagus nerve stimulation (VNS) and dietary approaches in CYPWE with ID (see Chapter 6), and surgical resection should not be discounted.

Unmet needs. It must also be remembered that epilepsy is one of the highest causes of preventable mortality and hospitalization for children and young people with ID.[28] The needs of this group were highlighted in 2014 in a White Paper sponsored by the ILAE and International Bureau for Epilepsy (IBE).[29] It outlines four domains requiring concerted international action:
- the development of standards and initiatives to enhance diagnosis, investigative pathways, and treatment
- guidelines for treatment, specifically best practice in the management of ASM

TABLE 7.1

Cognitive function associated with different epilepsy syndromes

Syndrome	Cognition and behavior
Self-limited focal epilepsies	
Self-limited epilepsy with centrotemporal spikes (SeLECTS)	Usually normal cognition; occasionally mild ID
Childhood occipital visual epilepsy (COVE)	Usually normal cognition; occasionally mild ID
Myoclonic epilepsy in infancy (MEI)	Normal cognition or mild ID (moderate to severe ID is rare); inattention and learning disorders may evolve over time
Generalized epilepsy syndromes	
Childhood absence epilepsy (CAE)	Usually normal cognition; some subtle learning difficulties and ADHD; rare in individuals with ID (other etiologies should be considered)
Juvenile myoclonic epilepsy (JME)	Usually normal cognition; sometimes impairment in specific cognitive domains such as executive function, attention, and decision-making; rare in individuals with mild ID; higher rates of impulsivity
Developmental and/or epileptic encephalopathies (DEE)	
Early infantile developmental and epileptic encephalopathy (EIDEE)	Moderate to severe ID (except those who receive early treatment for the underlying etiology)
Infantile epileptic spasms syndrome (IESS)	Severe ID (depends on etiology and promptness of treatment)
Dravet syndrome (DS)	Mild to severe ID; progressive cognitive decline; speech delay; behavior disorders; some inattention and hyperactivity

CONTINUED

TABLE 7.1 CONTINUED

Syndrome	Cognition and behavior
Lennox–Gastaut syndrome (LGS)	Moderate to severe ID in >90% of patients; behavior disorders such as hyperactivity, aggression, ASD, and sleep disturbances are common
DEE with spike-and-wave activation in sleep (DEE-SWAS)	Cognitive, behavioral, or psychiatric impairment; all cognitive domains are affected, including language and communication, temporospatial orientation, attention, and social interaction
Epilepsy with myoclonic-atonic seizures	Normal cognition or mild impairment; behavioral disorders, such as hyperactivity and aggression, and sleep disturbances improve or remit after seizure control
Hemiconvulsion-hemiplegia-epilepsy syndrome	Variable ID

Etiology-specific syndromes

Mesial temporal lobe epilepsy with hippocampal sclerosis (MTLE-HS)	Cognitive impairment with deficits in verbal memory (MTLE-HS that affects the dominant [usually left] lobe) or visual memory (MTLE-HS that affects the non-dominant temporal lobe)
Rasmussen syndrome	Progressive decline in cognition and language (the latter if the dominant hemisphere is affected)

ADHD, attention deficit hyperactivity disorder; ASD, autism spectrum disorder; ID, intellectual disability.
Adapted from Zuberi et al. 2022, Specchio et al. 2022, Riney et al. 2022, and Hirsch et al. 2022.[22–25]

- standards for primary care, multidisciplinary teamwork, and clinical consultations, with an emphasis on enhancing communication and access to information
- the enhancement of links across different stakeholders, organizations, and services.

Collaborative working is essential. Most services for people with ID do not have clinicians who possess an in-depth knowledge of neurology, while pediatricians and even pediatric neurologists are not usually well versed in the management of children and young people with ID. Close cooperation between services can minimize these shortfalls.

Further information on the treatment of individuals with ID and epilepsy is available in *Fast Facts: Epilepsy in Adults*.[30]

Sleep disturbances

Epilepsy has a bidirectional relationship with sleep.

In some epilepsies, seizures occur exclusively or predominantly during sleep, or interictal epileptogenic discharges may be activated during sleep.[31] Seizure frequency peaks at the start and end of sleep in primary GTCS, and sleep deprivation has been shown to increase seizure frequency. For example, in juvenile myoclonic epilepsy (JME) sleep deprivation has been shown to increase the frequency of both myoclonic and tonic-clonic seizures after waking; both the condition and its most effective treatment (sodium valproate) have been postulated to affect the circadian rhythm of children and young people with this syndrome.[32]

Epilepsy can also affect wakefulness. Epileptic discharges during sleep (either subclinical discharges or those that cause brief periods of arousal) can impair the restorative value or quality of sleep. In addition, as mentioned above, seizures may disrupt the circadian rhythm or reduce the overall amount of sleep. All these factors may affect daytime alertness and cause impairment in behavior or cognitive function.[33] To further complicate the picture, some medications such as phenytoin, phenobarbital, and benzodiazepines may negatively affect sleep architecture,[33] while perampanel may improve it.[34]

There can be confusion between epilepsy and sleep disorders and vice versa. This highlights the importance of good history taking and home video recordings to help to differentiate between seizures, parasomnias, and sleep disorders. If significant sleep disturbance persists or diagnostic doubt remains, video EEG or polysomnography may provide clarification.[33] Referral to a specialist sleep service should be considered, although the availability of these clinics can vary between regions.

If seizure control is poor, it is important to consider whether a comorbid sleep disorder such as obstructive sleep apnea (OSA) exists. Lack of normal sleep due to OSA may precipitate seizures, so if sleep apnea is a concern a referral should be made to an ear, nose, and throat specialist for appropriate assessment. Treatment for OSA has been shown to improve seizure control.[33]

If a child or young person with epilepsy is excessively sleepy or shows worsening behavior or cognition, it is worth considering a syndrome such as developmental and/or epileptic encephalopathy with spike-and-wave activation in sleep (DEE-SWAS).

Organizations such as The Sleep Charity (UK), National Sleep Foundation (USA), or Sleep Health Foundation (Australia) offer practical advice for improving sleep hygiene in children and young people (see Useful resources, page 183).

Cerebral palsy

Because of the underlying changes in the brain, 40–50% of individuals with cerebral palsy also have epilepsy, much higher than in the general population. Risk factors that increase the likelihood of children with cerebral palsy developing epileptic seizures include:

- major motor dysfunction (Gross Motor Function Classification System [GMFCS] IV–V), especially spastic quadriplegia-type presentations
- prematurity
- low birth weight
- neonatal seizures
- neonatal jaundice
- neonatal cyanosis.[35]

Children and young people with cerebral palsy are more likely to experience focal or focal to bilateral tonic-clonic seizures.[35] Epilepsy in children and young people with cerebral palsy is more frequently associated with polytherapy, refractory seizures, and long-term treatment with ASM.

Gastrointestinal and feeding problems

Gastrointestinal problems. CYPWE have a higher incidence of gastrointestinal problems than those without epilepsy. The most frequently reported are constipation and irritable bowel symptoms. For patients with drug-resistant epilepsy, periods of altered bowel movements have shown an association with increased seizure frequency. While there is limited clinical research in this area, preclinical studies have begun to look at the complex relationship between epilepsy and the microbiota-gut-brain axis.[36]

In the first instance, gastrointestinal issues should be managed by the child or young person's primary care provider, with referral to a gastroenterologist if issues persist.

Feeding difficulties. Children and young people with refractory epilepsy may be at higher risk of feeding difficulties, causing malnutrition. Feeding difficulties are more prevalent among CYPWE with significant disabilities. Chewing and swallowing difficulties, vomiting, and poor intake can be problematic for some CYPWE.[37] If there are concerns in these areas, referral to a speech and language therapist for an eating and drinking assessment, or to a dietician for a nutritional assessment, is advisable.

Bone health

CYPWE who take ASM may be at an increased risk of weak or breaking bones. Some ASM, such as sodium valproate and enzyme-inducing drugs such as carbamazepine, have a greater effect on bone health than others. However, all ASM are associated with lower vitamin D levels in pediatric patients.[38] The effects are greatest for CYPWE who have limited mobility and/or exposure to sunlight.

To ensure good bone health, CYPWE must have sufficient calcium (from yogurt, cheese, milk, etc.) and vitamin D (from sunlight, oily fish, red meat, liver, egg yolks, and some fortified foods) in their diet. In addition, if they are physically able, CYPWE should be encouraged to exercise regularly. CYPWE who have a limited diet, or who live in countries with periods of limited sunlight, should be advised to take a daily vitamin supplement that includes calcium and vitamin D.

Blood levels of calcium and vitamin D do not need to be measured routinely unless the child or young person shows symptoms of deficiency, they are at particularly high risk (for example, if they have low exposure to sunlight or are non-weight-bearing), or there is a clinical reason to do so (such as osteomalacia or a fall).[39]

Multidisciplinary support

Epilepsy, epileptic seizure activity, and the side effects of treatment may affect many areas of a child's or young person's life. It is therefore important that they receive holistic care, involving health professionals from a wide variety of disciplines, to minimize the effects of epilepsy on development and to maximize their potential.[40]

Education services and educational psychologist. As described above, CYPWE have a much higher incidence of ID than the general population. Areas such as memory and cognition may be affected by the underlying cause of the seizures, the seizure burden, or the side effects of medication. Early engagement, recognition, assessment, and support by education providers is important in understanding the challenges that CYPWE may be facing.

Clinical psychologist or local therapy services. As described above, CYPWE have a much higher incidence of mental health difficulties and suicide than their unaffected peers or children/young people with other chronic conditions, such as asthma and diabetes. CYPWE and their families need support to manage the psychosocial aspects of epilepsy.

Developmental pediatricians. Children with additional neurological difficulties have a much higher incidence of epilepsy than their neurotypical peers. Conversely, children with epilepsy have a higher incidence of conditions such ADHD and ASD. Early recognition and diagnosis of additional needs can increase the likelihood of accessing appropriate support.

Allied health professionals, such as speech and language therapists, occupational therapists, dietitians, and physiotherapists may be involved depending on the effect of epilepsy or comorbidities or complications.

Key points – comorbidities and complications

- When providing support for CYPWE it is important to consider how comorbidities may affect their diagnosis and how epilepsy may affect their comorbidities.
- CYPWE have higher rates of mental health issues, neurodiversity, and ID. Those who support them with their epilepsy can be essential in identifying concerns in these areas.
- Early identification of comorbid conditions and complications and referral to appropriate services can help to ensure that necessary support is put in place to maximize the potential of CYPWE.
- There is a significant relationship between sleep and seizures. It is therefore important to encourage good sleep hygiene in CYPWE, investigate any seizures that may be affecting sleep, or refer to an appropriate service if there are any concerns regarding sleep disorders.
- The adverse effects of some ASM, such as cognitive impairment or poor bone health, should be considered as part of the holistic care of CYPWE.
- Epilepsy care should be holistic, involving education, social, and healthcare providers, to minimize the effects of seizures, treatment, and comorbidities.

References

1. Davies S, Heyman I, Goodman R. A population survey of mental health problems in children with epilepsy. *Develop Med Child Neurol* 2003;45:292–5.

2. Heyman I, Skuse D, Goodman R. Brain disorders and psychopathology. In: *Rutter's Child and Adolescent Psychiatry*, 6th edn. Thapar A, Pine DS, Leckman JF et al., eds. Wiley-Blackwell, 2015.

3. Srinivas HV, Shah U. Comorbidities of epilepsy. *Neurol India* 2017;65(Supplement):S18–24.
4. Reilly C, Atkinson PA, Chin RF et al. Symptoms of anxiety and depression in school-aged children with active epilepsy: a population-based study. *Epilepsy Behav* 2015;52:174–9.
5. Reilly C, Agnew R, Neville BG. Depression and anxiety in childhood epilepsy: a review. *Seizure* 2011;20:589.
6. Wirrell EC, Bieber ED, Vanderwiel A et al. Self-injurious and suicidal behaviour in young adults, teens, and children with epilepsy: a population based study. *Epilepsia* 2020;61:1919–30.
7. Wagner JL, Kellermann T, Mueller M et al. Development and validation of the NDDI-E-Y: a screening tool for depressive symptoms in pediatric epilepsy. *Epilepsia* 2016;57:1265–70.
8. Coppola G, Operto FF, Matricardi S, Verrotti A. Monitoring and managing depression in adolescents with epilepsy: current perspectives. *Neuropsychiatr Dis Treat* 2019; 15:2273–80.
9. Walkup JT, Albano AM, Piacentini J et al. Cognitive behavioral therapy, sertraline, or a combination in childhood anxiety. *N Engl J Med* 2008;359:2753–66.

10. UCL Great Ormond Street Institute of Child Health. *The Mental Health Intervention for Children with Epilepsy (MICE) Project.* ucl.ac.uk/child-health/research/population-policy-and-practice-research-and-teaching-department/champp/psychological-7, last accessed 1 November 2023.
11. William AE, Giust JM, Kronenberger WG, Dunn DW. Epilepsy and attention-deficit hyperactivity disorder: links, risks, and challenges. *Neuropsychiatr Dis Treat* 2016;12:287–96.
12. National Institute for Health and Care Excellence (NICE). *Attention deficit hyperactivity disorder: diagnosis and management. NICE guideline [NG87].* NICE, 2018. nice.org.uk/guidance/ng87, last accessed 1 November 2023.
13. Stein MA, Weiss M, Hlavaty L. ADHD treatments, sleep, and sleep problems: complex associations. *Neurotherapeutics* 2012;9:509–17.
14. Sundelin HEK, Larsson H, Lichtenstein P et al. Autism and epilepsy. A population-based nationwide cohort study. *Neurology* 2016;87:192–7.
15. Hara H. Autism and epilepsy: a retrospective follow-up study. *Brain Develop* 2007;29:486–90.

Epilepsy in Children and Young People

16. Chez MG, Chang M, Krasne V et al. Frequency of epileptiform EEG abnormalities in a sequential screening of autistic patients with no known clinical epilepsy from 1996 to 2005. *Epilepsy Behav* 2006;8:267–71.

17. Freilinger M, Reisel B, Reiter E et al. Behavioural and emotional problems in children with epilepsy. *J Child Neurol* 2006;21:939–45.

18. Guifoyle SM, Follansbee-Junger K, Smith AW et al. Antiepileptic drug behavioural side effects and baseline hyperactivity in children and adolescents with new onset epilepsy. *Epilepsia* 2017; 59:146–54.

19. Tao S, Li J, Zhang M et al. The effects of mindfulness-based interventions on child and adolescent aggression: a systematic review and meta-analysis. *Mindfulness* 2021;12:1301–15.

20. Michaelis R, Tang V, Goldstein LH et al. Psychological treatments for adults and children with epilepsy: evidence-based recommendations by the International League Against Epilepsy Psychology Task Force. *Epilepsia* 2018;59:1282–302.

21. Robertson J, Hatton C, Emerson E, Baines S. Prevalence of epilepsy among people with intellectual disabilities: a systematic review. *Seizure* 2015;29:46–62.

22. Zuberi SM, Wirrell E, Yozawitz E et al. ILAE classification and definition of epilepsy syndromes with onset in neonates and infants: position statement by the ILAE Task Force on Nosology and Definitions. *Epilepsia* 2022;63:1349–97.

23. Specchio N, Wirrell EC, Scheffer IE et al. International League Against Epilepsy classification and definition of epilepsy syndromes with onset in childhood: position paper by the ILAE Task Force on Nosology and Definitions. *Epilepsia* 2022;63:1398–442.

24. Riney K, Bogacz A, Somerville E et al. International League Against Epilepsy classification and definition of epilepsy syndromes with onset at a variable age: position paper by the ILAE Task Force on Nosology and Definitions. *Epilepsia* 2022;63:1443–74.

25. Hirsch E, French J, Scheffer IE et al. ILAE definition of the idiopathic generalized epilepsy syndromes: position paper by the ILAE Task Force on Nosology and Definitions. *Epilepsia* 2022;63:1475–99.

26. Kim E-H, Ko T-S. Cognitive impairment in childhood onset epilepsy: up-to-date information about its causes. *Korean J Paediatr* 2016;59:155–64.

27. Shankar R, Mitchell S. *Step Together: Integrating Care for People with Epilepsy and a Learning Disability.* BILD 2020. bild.org.uk/wp-content/uploads/2020/11/Step-Together-17-November-2020-Download-Link-.pdf, last accessed 26 January 2024.

146

28. NHS. Learning Disability Mortality Review (LeDeR). *Action from Learning Report 2020/21*. University of Bristol, 2021. england.nhs. uk/publication/leder-action-from-learning-report-2021, last accessed 30 January 2024.

29. Kerr M, Linehan C, Thompson R et al. A White Paper on the medical and social needs of people with epilepsy and intellectual disability: the Task Force on Intellectual Disabilities and Epilepsy of the International League Against Epilepsy. *Epilepsia* 2014;55:1902–6.

30. Tittensor P, Shepley S, Brodie MJ. Specific populations: people with intellectual and developmental disabilities. In: *Fast Facts: Epilepsy in Adults*. S. Karger Publishers Ltd, 2023:142–54.

31. Stores G. Sleep disturbance in childhood epilepsy: clinical implications, assessment and treatment. *Arch Dis Child* 2013;98:548–51.

32. Xu L, Guo D, Liu YY et al. Juvenile myoclonic epilepsy and sleep. *Epilepsy Behav* 2018;80:326–30.

33. Nobili L, Beniczy S, Eriksson SH et al. Expert opinion: managing sleep disturbance in people with epilepsy. *Epilepsy Behav* 2021;124:1–12.

34. Rocamora R, Álvarez I, Chavarría B, Principe A. Perampanel effect on sleep architecture in patients with epilepsy. *Seizure* 2020;76:137–42.

35. Pavone P, Gulizia C, Le Pira A et al. Cerebral palsy and epilepsy in children: clinical perspectives on a common comorbidity. *Children (Basel)* 2020;8:16.

36. Federica A, Emanuele CI, Alessandra M et al. Functional gastrointestinal disorders in patients with epilepsy: reciprocal influence and impact on seizure occurrence. *Front Neurol* 2021;12:705126.

37. Bertoli S, Cardinali S, Veggiotti P et al. Evaluation of nutritional status in children with refractory epilepsy. *Nutr J* 2006;5:14.

38. Alhaidari HM, Babtain F, Alqadi F et al. Association between serum vitamin D levels and age in patients with epilepsy: a retrospective study from an epilepsy center in Saudi Arabia. *Ann Saudi Med* 2022;42:262–8.

39. McNamara NA, Romanowski EMF, Olson DP, Shellhaas RA. Bone health and endocrine comorbidities in pediatric epilepsy. *Semin Pediatr Neurol* 2017;24:301–9.

40. Goldstein J, Plioplys S, Zelko F et al. Multidisciplinary approach to childhood epilepsy: exploring the scientific rationale and practical aspects of implementation. *J Child Neurol* 2004;19:362–78.

**Neurology and
Neuroscience**

8 Getting older

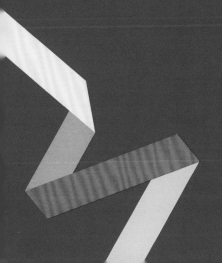

HEALTHCARE

Puberty and menstruation

All young people with epilepsy should receive individualized accurate advice and information about puberty, contraception, sexual relationships, and the importance of avoiding an unplanned pregnancy.

Effect on seizures. Changes to sex hormone levels during puberty can trigger seizures in some young people with epilepsy. Girls may find that their seizures worsen during their menstrual cycle, a phenomenon known as catamenial epilepsy. This exacerbation is thought to be a consequence of an imbalance between estrogen and progestogen concentrations. Hormonal preparations that induce amenorrhea can be successful in reducing catamenial epilepsy. Keeping a diary of menstrual cycles and seizure activity may help to optimize the use of an antiseizure medication (ASM) such as intermittent clobazam for the few days just before and shortly after the onset of menstruation.[1]

Treatment considerations. Girls with epilepsy should be offered effective contraception to avoid unplanned pregnancies. Hepatic enzyme-inducing ASM can cause some contraceptives to fail (Table 8.1; also see Chapter 5).[2] The metabolism of ASM can alter the menstrual cycle and increase turnover of the components of oral contraceptive pills (OCPs) and depot formulations of steroid hormones. To be effective, the combined OCP must provide at least 50 µg of estrogen/day. Medroxyprogesterone depot injections appear to be effective, and a levonorgestrel/copper intrauterine device (IUD) may also be an option. The progesterone-only pill, progesterone implant, combined contraceptive patches, and vaginal ring are not recommended as their effectiveness cannot be guaranteed.

For emergency contraception, a single dose of levonorgestrel, 3 mg, should be taken as soon as possible within 72 hours of unprotected intercourse. Ulipristal acetate is not recommended because of reduced efficacy; however, inserting a non-hormonal IUD within 5 days of intercourse is an alternative option.[2–4]

In general, OCPs do not reduce the efficacy of ASM. The exception is lamotrigine, and girls must be informed of this interaction. Any

TABLE 8.1

Hormonal contraceptive advice for girls with epilepsy taking enzyme-inducing antiseizure medication

Enzyme-inducing ASM	Recommendations	Not recommended	Additional information
CBZ CEN OXC PB PER (≥12 mg/day) PHT PRM RFN TPM (≥200 mg/day)	• Combined OCP must provide ≥50 µg/day of estrogen • If breakthrough bleeding with no other obvious cause, consider increasing estrogen to 70 µg/day, and tricycling • Seek guidance on dosage of combined OCP from the SmPC and latest editions of national formularies • Use depot/subcutaneous progesterone and levonorgestrel IUDs **Emergency contraception** • Single-dose levonorgestrel, 3 mg, as soon as possible within 72 hours of unprotected intercourse • Do not use ulipristal acetate; insert non-hormonal IUD within 5 days of intercourse instead • Ensure type and dose of emergency contraception is in line with the SmPC and latest editions of national formularies	• Progesterone-only pill • Progesterone implant • Combined contraceptive patches • Vaginal ring	• Discuss additional barrier methods, alternative oral contraception, or depot progestogen injections • Non-hormonal barrier methods are less effective than combined OCP; non-hormonal IUD may be contraceptive of choice • Risk of bone loss with depot/subcutaneous progesterone

ASM, antiseizure medication; CBZ, carbamazepine; CEN, cenobamate; IUD, intrauterine device; OCP, oral contraceptive pill; OXC, oxcarbazepine; PB, phenobarbital; PER, perampanel; PHT, phenytoin; PRM, primidone; RFN, rufinamide; SmPC, summary of product characteristics; TPM, topiramate. Adapted from Shepley 2016.[2]

estrogen-based contraceptive can cause a significant reduction in plasma concentrations of lamotrigine, resulting in loss of seizure control. Lamotrigine dose adjustment is usually required when a teenage girl starts taking these contraceptives. Progesterone-only contraceptives do not interact with lamotrigine and can be used without restriction. Girls with epilepsy taking other non-enzyme-inducing ASM (Table 8.2) should be informed that there is no known interaction with hormonal contraceptives.[2-4]

All teenage girls who are taking ASM and are at risk of unplanned pregnancy should take supplemental folic acid, 4–5 mg daily, to reduce the risk of neural tube defects.[5]

Sodium valproate is highly teratogenic. It carries a 10% risk of major congenital malformations and a 30–40% risk of neurodevelopmental, cognitive, and behavioral disorders following in utero exposure.[6] In the UK, no females of childbearing potential are prescribed sodium valproate unless other treatments are ineffective or not tolerated. Girls who have reached menarche and are taking sodium valproate must be entered into the Pregnancy Prevention Programme, which ensures they complete an annual risk acknowledgment form confirming that they have been informed of and understand the risks of using sodium valproate during pregnancy.[7] They must use highly effective contraception and see a specialist for review at least every year.

Medicines regulators around the world are also becoming concerned that sodium valproate could harm the children of men taking the drug. After a recent review of the available data, the UK's regulations are being strengthened to ensure that sodium valproate is not initiated in any new patients under the age of 55 (male or female) unless two independent specialists confirm that it is the most suitable treatment for that individual and there are no alternative options. Women and girls must continue to comply with the Pregnancy Prevention Programme.[7] Other medicines regulators are closely monitoring emerging data and it is likely that further regulatory controls will come into effect in other countries.

It is very important to inform girls that if they become pregnant they should not suddenly stop taking their ASM because of fear of causing harm to the unborn fetus. They need to contact their

TABLE 8.2

Hormonal contraceptive advice for girls with epilepsy taking non-enzyme-inducing antiseizure medication

Non-enzyme-inducing ASM	Recommendations
BRV	• As for girls not taking ASM
CLB	• Non-enzyme-inducing ASM do not alter the effectiveness of combined contraceptive patches, combined OCP, progesterone-only pill, progesterone implant, vaginal ring, or emergency contraceptives
CZP	
ESM	
LCM	
LEV	
PER (< 12 mg/day)	**Emergency contraception**
TGB	• As for girls not taking ASM
TPM	
VGB	
VPA	
ZNS	
LTG	• Progestogen-only contraceptives can be used without restriction
	• LTG clearance is doubled by ethinyl estradiol/levonorgestrel, 30 µg/150 µg, threatening seizure control; an increased LTG dose is usually required
	• Women should be made aware of signs and symptoms of LTG toxicity; the LTG dose should be reduced if these occur
	• Desogestrel may increase LTG concentrations
	Emergency contraception
	• As for girls not taking an ASM

ASM, antiseizure medication; BRV, brivaracetam; CLB, clobazam; CZP, clonazepam; ESM, ethosuximide; LCM, lacosamide; LEV, levetiracetam; LTG, lamotrigine; OCP, oral contraceptive pill; PER, perampanel; TGB, tigabine; TPM, topiramate; VGB, vigabatrin; VPA, sodium valproate; ZNS, zonisamide.
Adapted from Shepley 2016.[2]

primary care provider and/or usual epilepsy team. They also need to be informed about the risks associated with tonic-clonic seizures in pregnancy and the risk of sudden unexpected death in epilepsy (SUDEP). (See *Fast Facts: Epilepsy in Adults* for further information about preconception education, pregnancy, and postpartum management.[8])

Support at school

Stigma enacted by their peers can affect young people's ability to form relationships and develop their self-identity. Being bullied and isolated at school because of having epilepsy can negatively affect young people's quality of life and result in a lack of social interaction.[9] Young people with epilepsy may experience cognitive and memory disturbances secondary to seizures and side effects of ASM, both of which can have a negative effect on quality of life.[10] Despite not having an associated disability, epilepsy and seizures in young people with epilepsy may affect their learning and increase the risk of behavioral difficulties.[11]

Support at school is important for young people with epilepsy while they learn to negotiate and manage their condition and identity. In the UK, the 'Better Futures' campaign run by the National Centre for Young People with Epilepsy (NCYPE)[12] supports schools to develop practical formal training for teachers to:

- monitor achievement and behavior
- include young people in activities and provide a mentor
- liaise fully with parents and healthcare professionals
- be epilepsy aware and train to manage seizures.

Epilepsy charities and organizations can provide additional support to young people with epilepsy to help them achieve their maximum potential, for example by getting help at exam time and making decisions about further study and career choices (see Useful resources, page 183).

Important educational issues

Non-adherence to treatment. The importance of working with young people to improve adherence to ASM and reduce the risk of further seizures cannot be underestimated because of the increased risk of morbidity and mortality. As cognitive impairment can result in young people with epilepsy being forgetful, external memory aids, even something as simple as setting an alert on a mobile phone, may be helpful.

Drinking and drugs. Knowing the triggers for seizures can help young people with epilepsy learn how to modify their lifestyle to minimize the risk of occurrence. Alcohol and recreational drugs can lower the seizure threshold and cause and/or increase the frequency of seizures. Some prescribed medications can have a similar effect, and any healthcare professional advising on treatment for concomitant conditions must be made aware of the young person's epilepsy. Excess alcohol intake and recreational drugs should be avoided, and young people need to understand about the risk of SUDEP (see Chapter 1). Apps such as EpsMon (see page 158) are very useful ways of helping individuals to self-manage risk.

Disrupted sleep. Sleep deprivation and/or disturbed sleep can be a trigger for seizures (see page 140), so it is important for young people to report any sleep issues to their clinician. They should be advised to keep a regular sleep pattern and avoid late nights and drinking caffeine before bedtime. Some ASM such as lamotrigine can cause sleep disorders.[13] Anecdotally, these tend to manifest as insomnia and vivid dreams. Other ASM, such as perampanel, can improve sleep architecture, so alternative epilepsy treatments may help, alongside more traditional non-drug approaches.[14]

Mental health problems. The intrusive effect of seizures can affect all aspects of young people's lives. In a qualitative study, 63% of young people stated that, although they were happy much of the time, the unpredictability of seizures meant that most of them experienced periods of intense emotional distress. Other feelings included worry or fear (49%), sadness/dysphoria (45%), and anger/frustration (67%).[15]
Diagnosis of depression and risk of suicide in young people with epilepsy is inadequate and a more coordinated approach, which involves enabling young people and their families to recognize the signs of mental health problems early, cannot be underestimated (see page 130).[16]

Learning to drive. Young people with epilepsy may be able to apply for a driving license when they are of age. Regulations differ from country to country (and in the USA, Canada, and Australia, from state to state). Some countries, such as India, do not permit driving at all after an epilepsy diagnosis. In others, driving is permitted after seizure-free periods that vary from 6 to 36 months.[17]

In the EU and UK, driving is permitted 6 months after an isolated seizure, or after 12 months of seizure freedom if further episodes occur. In some countries, the seizure-free period depends on the seizure type. There are often special arrangements for people who only have seizures when they are asleep; they may be able to drive after a specified period, even if their sleep seizures continue.

The side effects of ASM, especially sedation, may interfere with a young person's ability to safely operate a vehicle, and advice should be given accordingly.

Overnight stays and travel. There should be no unnecessary restrictions to young people going on overnight stays and travel. Epilepsy charities and organizations provide advice and encourage young people to plan ahead and take particular precautions (Table 8.3).[18]

Transitioning to adult care

Transition in healthcare is the process in which professionals support young people to move successfully from childhood into adulthood. There can be a significant number of changes at this stage of a young person's life, not just in health but also in the education and social settings. Therefore, transition needs to adopt a person-centered approach.[19,20]

A young person with epilepsy may have been given their diagnosis in early childhood, at a time when they would not have been able to process the information needed to manage the condition in adulthood. This may include information about the diagnosis itself, treatment considerations, and lifestyle issues, such as those discussed in this chapter. Understanding potential triggers for seizures and how to minimize them is vital to reduce risk, up to and including that of SUDEP. SUDEP is a topic that also needs to be explored given that its incidence increases as young people approach adulthood, when there is less/no supervision and risk-taking behaviors increase.

Information needs to be individualized and tailored to the young person's age and level of cognitive ability. Easy-to-read literature may be required. Information also needs to be timely and given at

TABLE 8.3

Key travel advice for young people with epilepsy

- Avoid becoming overtired and dehydrated; if it is going to be a late night, try to sleep during the day
- Take your medication at regular intervals and make gradual adjustments to any time differences
- Check the expiry date of rescue medication for prolonged seizures and keep your medication with you at all times
- If travelling by plane, carry your medication in your hand luggage; the airline may want to know about your epilepsy diagnosis and what medication you are carrying, especially if it is in liquid form
- Carry a doctor's letter with information about your epilepsy and medication; if possible, have it translated into the language of the country you are travelling to
- Take medication in its original packaging and know its generic name, as the brand name may vary in different countries
- Ensure your travel insurance covers emergency medical treatment for epilepsy
- Wear a medical alert bracelet that includes your seizure details and an emergency contact number
- Take extra medication in case the return journey is delayed

Adapted from Young Epilepsy 2016.[18]

various stages during the transition process, beginning at around 13 years of age, with full handover to adult services happening at 16–18 years.[21] Topics will include practical information such as requesting prescriptions and obtaining benefits (in some countries, free prescriptions or travel passes may be available), opportunities for further education (support with studies is often offered by higher education institutions) and employment (certain jobs, particularly driving, flying, and serving in the armed forces will carry significant restrictions), and lifestyle choices (including the effects of alcohol, illicit and prescribed drugs, and sleep deprivation on seizure control). Informed decision-making during transition is important, with young people being encouraged to make good choices around treatment, sexual health, contraception, pregnancy, and their mental health.

For young people with a learning difficulty or disability there needs to be a focus on providing information to the young person's parents/ caregivers around the different situations that may arise in adulthood, including mental capacity, shared decision making (if the young person is unable to do this for themselves), and other legal aspects of healthcare within adult services.

Often the multidisciplinary team can support young people if they have complex medical needs. This will inevitably include more than one health discipline, meaning that close coordination between services is required to ensure the young person is successfully transitioned into adulthood. Continuity of care, a central coordinator, and patient-centered communication are essential for successful transition.[19]

Aids and tools

Self-management tools. A wealth of easy-to-read age-appropriate information is available in many formats from epilepsy charities and organizations (see Useful resources, page 183), which aim to help young people with epilepsy and their families learn about the condition and how to manage it. Resources include leaflets, factsheets, first aid posters, seizure care plans, and seizure diaries.[22]

Seizure care plans. There are many examples of seizure care plans available for self-completion and/or to complete with clinicians. Developing a care plan helps the young person with epilepsy make informed decisions about managing their condition, set goals, and have at least an annual review to discuss any issues that concern them.

Seizure diaries can be useful tools in clinical epilepsy reviews to monitor young people's epilepsy, including the types and duration of seizures, identify any specific triggers and patterns, and record any medication changes. Paper and electronic seizure diaries are freely available through epilepsy charities, and clinicians need to encourage young people with epilepsy to complete them.

There are also apps such as the multinational award-winning EpsMon (see Useful resources, page 183), which can help people with epilepsy monitor their seizure frequency and type and determine whether risks from seizures are worsening, improving, or staying the same. The app also helps CYPWE to record the risk factors mentioned above, including sleep disturbances, concomitant medication, alcohol, and stress. There are prompts to encourage positive action and, where necessary, review by a healthcare professional. The app should be revisited regularly and will prompt users to review their risks every 3 months.

Wearable devices such as wrist watches, armbands, and smartphones allow detection of motor seizure activity, alerting family members and caregivers in order for support to be provided. However, more research is needed to determine the effectiveness and reliability of most of these devices. Wearable devices capture changes in movement and/ or physiological signs but are not guaranteed to capture all seizure activity. No evidence has been found to determine whether non-EEG wearable devices can detect non-motor seizures,[22] nor if they can prevent SUDEP.[23]

Wrist-worn sensors are available to detect tonic-clonic seizures; information about these can be found on epilepsy charities' websites. Other wearable devices include fall alarms and alarms that people can carry on their person and activate when they need help. The use of wearable devices may improve the recording of seizures and response to ASM. It is very important that the young person with epilepsy and their family discuss the benefits and risks of wearable devices with their epilepsy team.

Non-wearable alarms and sensors can be equally important. These include epilepsy bed sensors, which can raise the alarm when young people have tonic-clonic seizures while asleep.

In all cases there are cost and subscription charges to consider.

Current early-stage research is focused on the possibility of developing a wearable device that can predict the risk of a seizure happening. The idea is to use artificial intelligence and machine learning to tailor such a device to an individual. Obvious challenges include determining the parameters that may be useful to provide advanced warning and which of these parameters it is possible to record.[24]

Medical identification cards and/or medical jewelry are very useful for young people with epilepsy to carry on their person in the event of a seizure while away from home. Vital information should include their name, date of birth, address, that they have epilepsy, type of seizures, medication, allergies, first aid information, and emergency contact numbers.

Key points – getting older

- All young people with epilepsy should receive individualized accurate advice and information about puberty, contraception, sexual relationships, and the importance of avoiding an unplanned pregnancy.
- Oral contraceptives containing at least 50 μg of estrogen should be used when co-administered with hepatic enzyme-inducing ASM, because these drugs induce metabolism of female sex hormones.
- Working with young people to improve adherence to medication is extremely important.
- Depression and anxiety are common in young people with epilepsy and have a significantly negative impact on quality of life.
- Young people with epilepsy should be supported at school, with teachers encouraging them to achieve their maximum potential.
- Young people with epilepsy should be counseled on lifestyle modifications that reduce the risk of provoking seizures without unduly limiting activities.
- Young people with epilepsy should be empowered and given tools for shared decision-making to self-manage their condition.

References

1. Frank S, Tyson NA. A clinical approach to catamenial epilepsy: a review. *Perm J* 2020;24:1–3.
2. Shepley SA. Preconception to postpartum care: the need to maximise the safety of women with epilepsy. *Br J Neurosci Nurs* 2016;12:3.
3. National Institute for Health and Care Excellence (NICE). *Epilepsies in children, young people and adults: diagnosis and management. NICE Guideline [NG217].* NICE, 2022. nice.org.uk/guidance/ng217, last accessed 1 November 2023.

4. Scottish Intercollegiate
Guidelines Network.
*Diagnosis and management of
epilepsy in adults: a national
clinical guideline.* Scottish
Intercollegiate Guidelines
Network, 2018. sign.ac.uk/
media/1079/sign143_2018.pdf,
last accessed 1 November 2023.

5. Kaplan YC, Koren G. Women
using antiepileptic drugs:
how much folic acid per day
is sufficient? *Motherisk Int J*
2020;1:22.

6. Medicines and Healthcare
products Regulatory Agency.
Medicines related to valproate:
risk of abnormal pregnancy
outcomes. GOV.UK, 2015.
gov.uk/drug-safety-update/
medicines-related-to-valproate-
risk-of-abnormal-pregnancy-
outcomes, last accessed
1 November 2023.

7. Medicines & Healthcare products
Regulatory Agency (MHRA).
*Valproate: review of safety data
and expert advice on management
of risks. Public assessment report.*
MHRA, 2023. assets.publishing.
service.gov.uk/media
/65660310312f400013e5d508
/Valproate-report-review-and-
expert-advice.pdf, last accessed
20 February 2024.

8. Tittensor P, Shepley S,
Brodie MJ. Specific populations:
pregnancy. In: *Fast Facts:
Epilepsy in Adults.* S. Karger
Publishers Ltd, 2023:135–40.

9. Lewis SA, Noyes J. Effective
process or dangerous precipice:
qualitative comparative
embedded case study with
young people with epilepsy
and their parents during
transition from children's to
adult services. *BMC Pediatr*
2013;13:169.

10. Kanner AM, Helmstaedter C,
Sadat-Hossieny Z, Meador K.
Cognitive disorders in
epilepsy I: clinical experience,
real-world evidence and
recommendations.
Seizure 2020;83:216–22.

11. Berg AT, Smith S, Frobish D
et al. Special education needs of
children with newly diagnosed
epilepsy. *Dev Med Child Neurol*
2005;47:749–53.

12. The National Centre for Young
People with Epilepsy (NCYPE).
The Better Futures Summit
25 March 2010. Summit Report
and Action Plan. NCYPE, 2010.
youngepilepsy.org.uk/sites/
default/files/dmdocuments/
CampaignHealthSummitReport.
pdf, last accessed 1 November
2023.

13. National Institute for Health
and Care Excellence (NICE).
*British National Formulary for
Children (BNFC).* NICE, 2023.
bnfc.nice.org.uk, last accessed
1 November 2023.

14. Rocamora R, Álvarez I,
Chavarría B, Principe A.
Perampanel effect on sleep
architecture in patients with
epilepsy. *Seizure* 2020;76:137–42.

15. Elliott I, Lach L, Smith M. I just want to be normal: a qualitative study exploring how children and adolescents view the impact of intractable epilepsy on their quality of life. *Epilepsy Behav* 2005;7:664–78.

16. Shafran R, Bennett S, Coughtrey A et al. Optimising evidence-based psychological treatment for the mental health needs of children with epilepsy: principles and methods. *Clin Child Fam Psychol Rev* 2020;23:284–95.

17. Ooi WW, Gutrecht JA. International regulations for automobile driving and epilepsy. *J Travel Med* 2000;7:1–4.

18. Young Epilepsy. Living with epilepsy: travelling and holidays. In: *Childhood Epilepsy. A Guide for Parents.* Young Epilepsy, 2016:34. youngepilepsy.org.uk/sites/default/files/dmdocuments/Childhood-epilepsy-A-Guide-for-Parents.pdf, last accessed 1 November 2023.

19. Goselink RJM, Olsson I, Malmgren K, Reilly C. Transition to adult care in epilepsy: a systematic review. *Seizure* 2022;101:52–9.

20. Camfield PR, Andrade D, Camfield C et al. How can transition to adult care be best orchestrated for adolescents with epilepsy? *Epilepsy Behav* 2019;93:138–47.

21. National Institute for Health and Care Excellence (NICE). *Epilepsies in children, young people and adults. Quality standard [QS211].* NICE, 2023. nice.org.uk/guidance/qs211, last accessed 24 January 2024.

22. Brinkmann BH, Karoly PJ, Nurse ES et al. Seizure diaries and forecasting with wearables: epilepsy monitoring outside the clinic. *Front Neurol* 2021;12:690404.

23. Jory C, Shankar R, Coker D et al. Safe and sound? A systematic literature review of seizure detection methods for personal use. *Seizure* 2016;36:4–15.

24. N-CODE. Can data from wearable technology predict when seizures will occur? Neuronostics Limited, 2023. N-code.org/wp-content/uploads/2023/02/NCODEproposal_Wearables_2023_nonconf.pdf, last accessed 20 June 2023.

9 Emergency care

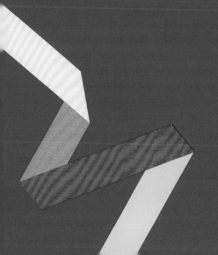

HEALTHCARE

Status epilepticus

Status epilepticus (SE) is a life-threatening emergency characterized by frequent and/or prolonged seizures. It is the most common neurological emergency of childhood. The incidence is approximately 20 cases per 100 000 children per year.[1] Although all seizure types can manifest as SE, the most readily recognized are prolonged or multiple, convulsive, tonic-clonic seizure(s).

There are two significant time points, which vary according to seizure type.

- T_1 is reached when a seizure is unlikely to self-terminate
  - 5 minutes for generalized tonic-clonic seizures (GTCS)
  - 10 minutes for focal seizures with impaired consciousness
  - 10–15 minutes for absence SE (although evidence for this is limited).
- T_2 is when neuronal injury can occur
  - 30 minutes for GTCS
  - more than 60 minutes for focal seizures with impaired consciousness.

Operationally, T_2 is considered to have been reached if a tonic-clonic seizure(s) lasts for 30 minutes from onset.[2,3]

Convulsive SE can lead to significant cognitive and behavioral impairments later in life. More serious are the immediate physiological effects, including hypertension, cardiac arrhythmias, tachycardia, and hyperthermia, with a mortality rate of 1.3–3.5% in children and young people, compared with 6.9–29.6% in adults.[4]

Early recognition of seizures and effective early pharmacological management can help to prevent SE. Therefore, a robust, succinct plan of management for parents, caregivers, and education staff is required to administer prehospital treatment.

Emergency care in the community

Standard first aid. When a child or young person experiences a tonic-clonic seizure, they should be protected from injury by cushioning their head and removing any objects that may cause injury to limbs. When the convulsive part of the seizure has stopped, the individual should be placed in a semiprone position with their head down (recovery position) to prevent aspiration. The seizure should be timed from the onset and the first aider should stay to reassure the child or young person until recovery.

Emergency first aid. When a child or young person with or without epilepsy experiences their first prolonged tonic-clonic seizure, lasting more than 5 minutes, and/or repeated tonic-clonic seizures in the community, standard first aid should be administered (as above) and the emergency services should be called immediately for early intervention.

Some CYPWE who have experienced SE previously should have rescue antiseizure medication (ASM) and an agreed individualized epilepsy treatment plan for family, caregivers, and education staff to follow (see below). Once rescue ASM is administered the child or young person should be monitored carefully for signs of recovery.[5]

Parents, caregivers, and education staff should be trained by a healthcare professional to provide first aid, administer rescue medication, and recognize side effects such as excessive sedation, amnesia, and confusion.[6] Administration of rescue ASM is usually limited to one dose in the community, because of the risks of respiratory depression.

The first aider must call emergency services if a rescue ASM is not effective within 10 minutes of administering the dose (or sooner according to education policy in schools), or if the child or young person is experiencing breathing difficulties or has sustained any injuries. Parents, caregivers, and education staff should also be advised not to repeat the dose within 24 hours, unless directed by their medical team.

Rescue medication. ASM for SE include oromucosal/intranasal midazolam, rectal diazepam, rectal paraldehyde, and, in a few countries, oromucosal lorazepam.

In the community setting, benzodiazepines such as oromucosal midazolam and rectal diazepam are the first and second-line ASM rescue treatment for SE. The use of rescue medication at the right time and for the right purpose can significantly improve outcomes. In the UK, best practice guidelines have been developed for the administration of oromucosal midazolam in the community.[7,8]

Oromucosal treatment. In some countries, oromucosal midazolam is available in prefilled syringes containing different doses depending on the child's age and bodyweight: 2.5 mg, 5 mg, 7.5 mg, and 10 mg. Alternatively, caregivers may need to draw up the required amount from a bottle or glass vial using a syringe (see page 94).

Rectal treatment. Rectal diazepam is available in 2.5 mg, 5 mg, and 10 mg doses, and is used if oromucosal/intranasal midazolam is contraindicated or unavailable (see page 84).

Rectal paraldehyde can be given as first-line treatment for SE if the child or young person has previously experienced respiratory depression after the administration of benzodiazepines. It is safe and effective to use with no reported effects of respiratory depression. The dose is dependent on the bodyweight of the child or young person (see page 96). However, administration can be challenging, as there are no preprepared administration systems and the drug dissolves plastics and rubber, meaning that it must be used within 15 minutes of the dose being prepared.

Training. Once a child or young person has been prescribed rescue medication, education and training should be provided to anyone involved in the care of that individual, including parents, caregivers, support staff, and teachers. Information should be provided on basic first aid for seizures, including how to position the child or young person during a seizure, non-administration of drinks/food during the seizure, monitoring of breathing and color, noting the time the seizure started or was first witnessed, when to seek medical help, remaining with the child or young person until help arrives, and how to administer the rescue medication.[7,8] Resuscitation training should also be offered and provided to parents in case a benzodiazepine has to be administered.

Emergency care in the hospital

In the hospital setting, intravenous lorazepam is first-choice treatment for SE (see page 94). However, it is often used as a second-line drug if a single dose of rectal diazepam or oromucosal/intranasal midazolam has been ineffective in stopping the seizure before the patient reaches hospital. In some countries, oromucosal lorazepam preparations are available as an alternative to midazolam. No more than two doses of a benzodiazepine should be administered outside a hospital setting due to the risk of respiratory depression. If the seizure persists in hospital despite two doses of benzodiazepines, intravenous ASM should be started. Evidence for the choice of treatment in children is limited, but phenytoin, levetiracetam, and sodium valproate are all reasonable options. Levetiracetam is preferred as it is quicker to administer with fewer adverse effects.

If the seizure persists for more than 60 minutes, the individual is considered to have developed refractory SE and general anesthesia may be warranted, alongside intravenous ASM such as phenytoin, sodium valproate, or levetiracetam.[9]

The International League Against Epilepsy (ILAE) has produced a pocket card of an algorithm for first-, second-, and third-line treatment options in managing SE (see Useful resources, page 183).

Epilepsy management plan

Epilepsy management plans should be individualized and provide relevant succinct information. There is no set format for an individual healthcare plan for epilepsy, but input should be obtained from healthcare professionals, education staff, parents/caregivers and, if possible, the child or young person to produce the plan. The charity Epilepsy Action has devised a prompt sheet to help gather the relevant information to produce an individual healthcare plan that includes details of the seizure(s) and/or epilepsy syndrome and seizure triggers, the action to be taken before, during, and after a seizure, the recommended treatment, any specific difficulties the child or young person needs help with (for example, learning, behavioral, or emotional problems), and details of the available support (see Useful resources, page 183).

The healthcare plan should be reviewed on at least a yearly basis or if the individual's condition, seizure pattern, or management of prolonged seizures change.

Key points – emergency care

- SE is a life-threatening medical emergency.
- In the community, SE treatment needs to be administered by parents, caregivers, and education staff who have been sufficiently trained with an understanding of epilepsy awareness and safe administration of rescue medication.
- If the seizure persists for more than 60 minutes, the child or young person is considered to have developed refractory SE.
- Individual healthcare plans need to be relevant and succinct documents that highlight the individual needs of the child in conjunction with the wishes of the family.

References

1. Gurcharran K, Grinspan ZM. The burden of pediatric status epilepticus: epidemiology, morbidity, mortality, and costs. *Seizure* 2019;68:3–8.

2. International League Against Epilepsy (ILAE). Time is brain: treating status epilepticus. Epigraph vol. 20, issue 2, Fall 2018 [online]. ILAE, 2018. ilae.org/journals/epigraph/epigraph-vol-20-issue-2-fall-2018/time-is-brain-treating-status-epilepticus, last accessed 1 November 2023.

3. Trinka E, Cock H, Hesdorffer D et al. A definition and classification of status epilepticus – report of the ILAE Task Force on Classification of Status Epilepticus. *Epilepsia* 2015;56:1515–23.

4. Lu M, Faure M, Bergamasco A et al. Epidemiology of status epilepticus in the United States: a systematic review. *Epilepsy Behav* 2020;112:107459.

5. National Institute for Health and Care Excellence (NICE). *Epilepsies in children, young people and adults. NICE guideline [NG217]*. NICE, 2022. nice.org.uk/guidance/ng217, last accessed 1 November 2023.

6. Dumeier HK, Neininger MP, Bernhard MK et al. Knowledge and attitudes of school teachers, preschool teachers and students in teacher training about epilepsy and emergency management of seizures. *Arch Dis Child* 2015;100:851–5.

7. Tittensor P, Tittensor S, Chisanga E et al. UK framework for basic epilepsy training and oromucosal midazolam administration. *Epilepsy Behav* 2021;122:108180.

8. Epilepsy Nurses Association (ESNA). The use of buccal midazolam. Best practice guidelines for training professional carers in the administration of buccal (oromucosal) midazolam for the treatment of prolonged and/ or clusters of epileptic seizures in the community. ESNA, Royal College of Psychiatrists, International League Against Epilepsy (British Branch), 2019. esna-online.org/wp-content/ uploads/2018/12/June-2019-Midazolam-guidelines.pdf, last accessed 1 November 2023.

9. National Institute for Health and Care Excellence (NICE). 7: Treating status epilepticus, repeated or cluster seizures, and prolonged seizures. In: *Epilepsies in children, young people, and adults. NICE guideline [NG217]*. NICE, 2022. nice.org.uk/guidance/ng217/ chapter/7-Treating-status-epilepticus-repeated-or-cluster-seizures-and-prolonged-seizures, last accessed 1 November 2023.

Further reading

Bellon M, Pfeiffer W, Maurici V. Choice and control: how involved are people with epilepsy and their families in the management of their epilepsy? Results from an Australian survey in the disability sector. *Epilepsy Behav* 2014;37:227–32.

Henshaw P. Managing epilepsy in the school environment. *Br J School Nurs* 2019;14:278–82.

Johnson EC, Atkinson P, Muggeridge A et al. Epilepsy in schools: views on educational and therapeutic provision, understanding of epilepsy and seizure management. *Epilepsy Behav* 2021;122:108179.

Luff E. Seizures: management in children. *Br J Child Health* 2020;1:20–5.

Penovich P, Glauser T, Becker D et al. Recommendations for development of acute seizure action plans (ASAPs) from an expert panel. *Epilepsy Behav* 2021;123:108264.

Pickering C. Epilepsy: recognition and management of seizures in children and young people. *Br J Child Health* 2021;2:136–42.

Rowland AG, Gill AM, Stewart AB et al. Review of the efficacy of rectal paraldehyde in the management of acute and prolonged tonic-clonic convulsions. *Arch Dis Child* 2009;94:720–3.

Sasidaran K, Singhi S, Singhi P. Management of acute seizure and status epilepticus in pediatric emergency. *Indian J Pediatr* 2012;79:510–17.

Trinka E, Leitinger M. Management of status epilepticus, refractory status epilepticus, and super-refractory status epilepticus. *Continuum (Minneap Minn)* 2022;28:559–602.

Neurology and
Neuroscience

10 Functional seizures

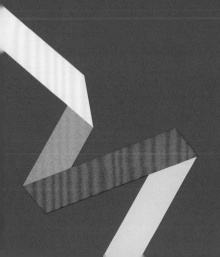

HEALTHCARE

Functional seizures, also termed dissociative seizures, non-epileptic attack disorder (NEAD), psychogenic non-epileptic seizures, and commonly (though most unhelpfully) the pejorative name pseudoseizures, are observable abrupt paroxysmal changes in behavior or consciousness that resemble epileptic seizures. They are a diagnostic challenge for the epilepsy clinician, especially in the teenage population.

Epidemiology
In contrast to functional seizures in adults, there is no female predominance in children and young people.[1] Seizures can present in children as young as 5 years old; however, studies indicate that the mean age of presentation in children and young people ranges from 10.5 to 14.2 years.[2]

Triggers
Functional seizures are regarded as a conversion disorder. Various biopsychosocial factors predispose patients to the condition and precipitate episodes, while others perpetuate the condition (Figure 10.1).[3] Predisposing risk factors for pediatric functional seizures include physical or sexual abuse (though these are less commonly reported than in adults), and school phobia or difficulties, including bullying, learning difficulties, and unrealistic expectations.[4] A study of children aged 6–16 years found that medical comorbidities, such as asthma, nocturnal enuresis, and chronic poor health, could also induce functional seizures.[5] Furthermore, children with pre-existing psychological/psychiatric diagnoses, epilepsy, head injury, and other brain pathology have been shown to be at higher risk of developing functional seizures.

Diagnosis
Clinical and psychosocial features of functional seizures in children and young people differ from those in the adult population. A mixed semiology of gross motor movements followed by minor motor movements in a repeating pattern, progressing to tremoring, falls, and an aura toward the end, contrasts with the rhythmic shaking or 'swooning' attacks commonly seen in adults. Motor inhibition is more common than hypermotor events in children and young people.[6]

The duration of functional seizures is often much longer than epileptic seizures. Functional seizures can be serial, with or without

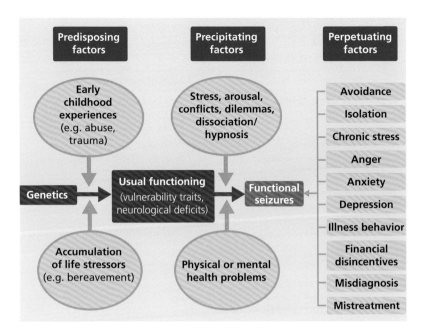

Figure 10.1 Predisposing, precipitating, and perpetuating biopsychosocial aspects of functional seizures. Adapted from Voon et al. 2016.[3]

full awareness returning in between attacks. Status epilepticus (SE), with repeated seizures, is unusual in people with established epilepsy. Therefore, reports of serial seizures over many minutes, or occasionally hours, should be red flags for functional seizures, particularly when this is the habitual pattern.

Similarly, recovery phases can be very different from those expected in epilepsy. Typically, children and young people with epilepsy (CYPWE) become orientated and coherent very quickly after a seizure, though they may be tired for a prolonged period afterward. Conversely, some people recover much more slowly from a functional seizure than would be expected in epilepsy.

Table 10.1 summarizes the clinical signs of epilepsy versus functional seizures.[7,8]

History taking. The level of diagnostic certainty for functional seizures is heavily reliant on the quality of witness history and the

TABLE 10.1

Differentiation of epileptic and functional seizures

	Level of evidence
Signs that favor functional seizures	
Long duration	Good
Fluctuating course	Good
Asynchronous movements	Good (frontal lobe focal seizures excluded)
Pelvic thrusting	Good (frontal lobe focal seizures excluded)
Side-to-side head or body movement	Good (convulsive events only)
Closed eyes	Good
Ictal crying	Good
Memory recall	Good
Signs that favor epileptic seizures	
Occurrence during sleep (EEG confirmed)	Good
Postictal confusion	Good
Stertorous breathing	Good (convulsive events only)
Other signs	
Gradual onset	Insufficient
Non-stereotyped events	Insufficient
Flailing or thrashing movements	Insufficient
Opisthotonus/'arc de cercle'	Insufficient
Tongue biting	Insufficient
Urinary incontinence	Insufficient

Adapted from Avbersek and Sisodiya 2010.[8]
PNES, psychogenic non-epileptic seizures.

experience of the clinician. It is important to examine the language used by the child or young person and their parents to describe the seizures. People with epilepsy usually try to carefully describe the physical event, whereas people with functional seizures tend to describe the consequences of the seizure.[9] On direct questioning,

CYPWE may describe being aware but unable to respond to those around them during the seizure. Useful questions to ascertain this include:

• Can you hear mum and dad asking if you are OK?
• Can you describe what it feels like inside your body?

Positive answers to these questions during a convulsive seizure may suggest functional seizures. However, it is important to ensure that the child or young person is describing awareness during the seizure, rather than before or after the seizure.

It is very important to establish timeframes for each section of the event, particularly the postictal phase. Witnesses should be asked whether the individual's eyes were open, closed, or rapidly blinking. If they were opened by someone else, it is important to ascertain if they closed as soon as the eyelid was released. Seizures due to epilepsy occur with the eyes open: anything different should be a clear red flag for functional seizures.

If the episode was convulsive, the nature of the movements should be determined. It can be helpful to mime. Useful questions to ask include:

• Was the child jerking, or was the movement more tremulous, as if they were very cold?
• Did the shaking stop abruptly, did it stop and re-start, or did it wax and wane in intensity?

The jerks usually become bigger and slower toward the end of generalized tonic-clonic seizures (GTCS).

Telemetry. Video recordings can be extremely helpful in differentiating functional from epileptic seizures, but recording a habitual episode with video EEG remains the gold standard diagnostic tool. Of course, this is dependent upon the seizures being relatively frequent and the child or young person accepting a period of telemetry. In practice, this limits the scope for conclusive diagnostic testing. Indeed, the length of time from onset to diagnosis can be measured in months to years.[10]

Diagnostic criteria. The rule of two can be helpful: at least two normal EEGs, with at least two seizures per week and resistance to two antiseizure medications (ASM) give an 85% positive predictive value for functional seizures.[7] An uncertain diagnosis has major implications for the management and treatment of functional seizures – diagnostic doubt is often associated with a poor prognosis.[7]

Management

It is vital that the diagnosing clinician spends time providing reassurance and clearly explaining the condition and the treatment options (Table 10.2).[11] This may need a much longer appointment than would be necessary in epilepsy, particularly as the explanation needs to be tailored to the age of the child or young person, taking into account any learning difficulties they may have. A clear explanation, particularly when the diagnosis has been made quickly and the child or young person has ongoing support, can render some individuals seizure free without more intensive treatment.

It is important to acknowledge that the seizures are real, and not in some way put on, and that while they are not as dangerous as epileptic seizures, people can and do suffer injuries because of them.

Management challenges. There are no standardized assessments or decision-making tools for the management of functional seizures. In one study, a standardized questionnaire was given to 66 doctors at a child and adolescent psychiatry conference. Two-thirds of the respondents felt that local services for treating people with functional seizures were poorly managed. For example, 20% of children without epilepsy were still being treated with an ASM 6 months after receiving their diagnosis of functional seizures.[12]

All too frequently, patients are given reassurances, ASM is no longer prescribed, and some relatively low-level psychological support may be offered. Children with a co-existing diagnosis of epilepsy may receive psychological support. However, for children and young people with a diagnosis of functional seizures alone, psychological input is woefully under-resourced in developed health economies, and completely lacking in the developing world.[6]

Improving outcomes. A structured plan involving the multidisciplinary team and a named primary point of contact for the patient (depending on the service, this could be a pediatric epilepsy specialist nurse, pediatric neurologist, pediatric neuropsychiatrist, or

TABLE 10.2

Strategies for communicating the diagnosis of functional seizures

Most useful concepts	Example language
Explain what functional seizures are not (i.e. epilepsy) but acknowledge that it is still possible for the seizures to cause injury	Good news, the seizures are not caused by epilepsy and therefore you don't need to take ASM. The seizures are less dangerous, but they can still cause injury.
Reassure that the seizures are real	These seizures happen at a subconscious level. You are not crazy. The seizures can be frightening and disabling, and can sometimes cause injury. You are not putting them on.
Give a name to the condition	These seizures have many different names. We prefer functional or dissociative seizures, or non-epileptic attack disorder, but you might hear terms like psychogenic non-epileptic seizures or pseudoseizures, which some people with this condition do not like.
Explain that functional seizures are common	We see lots of people with these kinds of seizures. There are support groups, many of which are online via social media.
Explain what functional seizures are	Seizures can be related to stress, emotion, difficult thoughts, and memories. It is possible to get into a vicious cycle where there is worry or stress leading to more seizures which leads to more stress. It can be hard to pinpoint triggers. Some people have a history of psychological trauma or abuse, but this isn't always the case. [Patients will often read about this, so it's almost always better to bring it up during the consultation.]
Withdrawal of ASM (if prescribed). The precise timing will depend on the confidence of the individual	We need to withdraw your medication gradually to avoid side effects.

CONTINUED

TABLE 10.2 CONTINUED

Strategies for communicating the diagnosis of functional seizures

Most useful concepts	Example language
Reassurance of support. Ensure the patient knows who to contact for advice between appointments	We will continue with follow-up appointments here, but psychology/psychiatry referral will also be helpful.
Discuss treatment options. Seizures sometimes stop after a clear explanation. When they do not, psychological treatments are helpful. Discuss what is available in your area and describe basic concepts of interventions like CBT	Although tablets don't help your seizures, several very effective talking therapies are available. [Precisely what the clinician then talks about will depend on the availability of services locally, but may include CBT, acceptance commitment therapy, mindfulness, or relaxation. Current thinking suggests that there is not a 'one-size-fits-all' approach, so an option to try various treatments is important.]

ASM, antiseizure medication; CBT, cognitive behavioral therapy.
Adapted from LaFrance et al. 2013.[11]

pediatric psychiatric nurse) would undoubtedly improve outcomes. A stepwise holistic approach, recognizing the patient as an individual and accepting that no single treatment will work for everyone, should be the overarching principle of management.

Given that access to expert psychological treatment is limited, it is very important that the diagnosing team remains involved to signpost the individual to relevant services and resources, unless a more appropriate service is available locally.

Psychological treatment. No single psychological treatment will work for everyone with functional seizures. Cognitive behavioral therapy (CBT) is the approach with most evidence, though a large multicenter trial (CODES) failed to demonstrate an overall reduction in seizures.[13] Secondary outcome measures showed significant improvements in overall health, and this principle of seeing seizures as a symptom of another underlying problem is a key concept in successful management.

Addressing triggers, which could be physical (particularly pain) or emotional may be the best way forward. Given that issues around school, such as unrealistic expectations of parents, bullying, or social adjustment, are common triggers, a multidisciplinary approach involving education can be helpful.

That isn't to say that direct intervention aimed at aborting seizures can't be effective. Grounding techniques can be extremely useful if the child or young person has a seizure warning. Individuals can learn to modify their lifestyle in response to seizure triggers, in the same way that life hygiene principles can be useful in epilepsy. However, care needs to be taken to limit avoidance behavior, which can have a significant detrimental effect, causing social isolation and worsening seizures.

Acceptance commitment therapy (ACT) has been studied in epilepsy. While there is no evidence from large-scale trials for the use of this technique in people with functional seizures, the principles underpinning ACT, particularly mindfulness, can be hugely beneficial, and there is evidence citing its usefulness in a pediatric population.[14] Explaining the principle of treating the individual and their underlying diagnosis rather than purely counting seizures is a very helpful approach.

Other management options. Several studies have suggested that relaxation techniques can be helpful in treating epileptic seizures, and it is certainly possible that these techniques could also be useful for some individuals with functional seizures. Aromatherapy, with or without hypnosis, may have a place here too. Self-help techniques are described in detail at nonepilepticattacks.info.

Brief, manualized, psychoeducational interventions delivered by non-psychologists can also be helpful, though the data are mixed.[15] Small case studies have reported improvements in functional seizures with eye movement desensitization and reprocessing (EMDR).[16]

Group therapy and family therapy can be helpful for some people, as can anger and anxiety management courses.

Key points – functional seizures

- Functional seizures are one of the most challenging differential diagnoses for pediatricians evaluating possible seizures in children and young people; the term is used to denote the distinction between epileptic seizures and medically unexplained seizures.
- There are important differences in the cause of functional seizures in children and young people, with an emphasis on problems with school and interpersonal relationships rather than abuse.
- Functional seizures fall into the broad category of motor inhibition and motor attacks, with the former being more common in children while the latter are more usual in adults.
- The level of diagnostic certainty for functional seizures depends heavily on the quality of witness history and clinician experience.
- Home video recordings of paroxysmal events can be helpful for differential diagnosis.
- A clear explanation of functional seizures following a rapid diagnosis, and with ongoing support, can lead to some people becoming seizure free without more intensive treatment.
- The treatment of functional seizures in children and young people has a different emphasis from adults and often requires multidisciplinary management, working with educationalists and pediatric mental health clinicians.
- Pharmacological treatment of functional seizures is only indicated if there is a treatable underlying trigger such as anxiety, depression, migraine, or pain.

References

1. Bompaire F, Barthelemy S, Monin J et al. PNES epidemiology: what is known, what is new? *Eur J Trauma Dissociation* 2021;5:100136.
2. Operto FF, Coppola G, Mazza R et al. Psychogenic nonepileptic seizures in pediatric population: a review. *Brain Behav* 2019; 9:e01406.
3. Voon V, Cavanna AE, Coburn K et al. Functional neuroanatomy and neurophysiology of functional neurological disorders (conversion disorder). *J Neuropsychiatry Clin Neurosci* 2016; 28:168–90.
4. Yeom JS, Bernard H, Koh S. Myths and truths about pediatric psychogenic nonepileptic seizures. *Clin Exp Pediatr* 2021;64:25159.
5. Madaan P, Gulati S, Chakrabarty B et al. Clinical spectrum of psychogenic non epileptic seizures in children; an observational study. *Seizure* 2018;59:60–6.
6. Kanemoto K, LaFrance WC Jr, Duncan R et al. PNES around the world: where we are now and how we can close the diagnosis and treatment gaps – an ILAE PNES Task Force report. *Epilepsia Open* 2017;2:307–16.
7. LaFrance WC Jr, Baker GA, Duncan R et al. Minimum requirements for the diagnosis of psychogenic nonepileptic seizures: a staged approach: a report from the International League Against Epilepsy Nonepileptic Seizures Task Force. *Epilepsia* 2013;54:2005–18.
8. Avbersek A, Sisodiya S. Does the primary literature provide support for clinical signs used to distinguish psychogenic nonepileptic seizures from epileptic seizures? *J Neurol Neurosurg Psychiatry* 2010;81:719–25.
9. Plug L, Sharrack B, Reuber M. Conversation analysis can help to distinguish between epilepsy and non-epileptic seizure disorders: a case comparison. *Seizure* 2009;18:43–50.
10. Caplan R, Doss J, Plioplys S, Jones JE. Diagnosis of pediatric PNES. In: *Pediatric Psychogenic Non-Epileptic Seizures*. Springer, 2017:3–14.
11. LaFrance WC Jr, Reuber M, Goldstein LH. Management of psychogenic nonepileptic seizures. *Epilepsia* 2013;54:53–67.
12. McWilliams A, Reilly C, Heyman I. Nonepileptic seizures in children: views and approaches at a UK child and adolescent psychiatry conference. *Seizure* 2017;53:23–5.
13. Goldstein LH, Robinson EJ, Meller JDC, Stone J. Cognitive behavioural therapy for adults with dissociative seizures (CODES): a pragmatic, multicentre, randomised controlled trial. *Lancet* 2020; 7:491–505.
14. Swain J, Hancock K, Dixon A, Bowman J. Acceptance and commitment therapy for children: a systematic review of intervention studies. *J Contextual Behav Sci* 2015;4:73–85.

15. Mayor R, Brown RJ, Cock H et al. A feasibility study of a brief psycho-educational intervention for psychogenic nonepileptic seizures. *Seizure* 2013;22:760–5.

16. Cope SR, Mountford L, Smith JG, Agrawal N. EMDR to treat functional neurological disorder: a review. *J EMDR Practice Res* 2018;12:118–31.

Further reading

Cope S, Poole N, Agrawal N. Treating functional non-epileptic attacks – should we consider acceptance and commitment therapy? *Epilepsy Behav* 2017;73: 197–203.

Hall-Patch L, Brown R, House A et al. Acceptability and effectiveness of a strategy for the communication of the diagnosis of psychogenic nonepileptic seizures. *Epilepsia* 2010;51:70–8.

Useful resources

Professional organizations

American Academy of Neurology
aan.com

American Epilepsy Society
aesnet.org

Association of British Neurologists
theabn.org

Association for Contextual
Behavioral Science
contextualscience.org

British Paediatric Neurology
Association
bpna.org.uk

Paediatric Epilepsy Training (PET)
courses
courses.bpna.org.uk/index.
php?page=paediatric-epilepsy-training

International Bureau for Epilepsy
ibe-epilepsy.org

International League Against Epilepsy
ilae.org

ilae.org/guidelines/guidelines-
and-reports

ilae.org/files/dmfile/StatusEpilepticus_
pocket_card.pdf

epilepsydiagnosis.org
(online diagnostic manual)

Epilepsy Nurses Association (ESNA)
esna-online.org

National Institute for Health and Care
Excellence (UK)
nice.org.uk
Guidelines
nice.org.uk/guidance/ng217

Scottish Intercollegiate Guidelines
Network
sign.ac.uk

Guidelines
sign.ac.uk/media/1844/sign-159-
epilepsy-in-children-final.pdf

sign.ac.uk/patient-and-public-
involvement/patient-publications/
epilepsy-in-children

Patient organizations

Brainwave (UK)
brainwave.org.uk

Canadian Epilepsy Alliance
canadianepilepsyalliance.org

Epilepsy Action (UK)
epilepsy.org.uk

Prompt sheet for indvidual healthcare plan
epilepsy.org.uk/app/uploads/2022/06/
ihp_prompt_questions.pdf

Epilepsy Foundation (USA)
epilepsy.com

Epilepsy Society (UK)
epilepsysociety.org.uk

FND Action (UK)
fndaction.org.uk

FND Guide UK
neurosymptoms.org

Matthew's Friends (UK)
Information about ketogenic dietary
therapies
matthewsfriends.org

National Sleep Foundation (USA)
thensf.org

The Sleep Charity (UK)
thesleepcharity.org.uk

Sleep Foundation (USA)
sleepfoundation.org

Sleep Health Foundation (Australia)
sleephealthfoundation.org.au

SUDEP Action (UK)
sudep.org

EpSMon: Epilepsy Self-Monitoring
sudep.org/epilepsy-self-monitor

Very Well Mind
verywellmind.com/what-is-the-misinformation-effect-2795353

Young Epilepsy (UK)
youngepilepsy.org.uk

FastTest

You've read the book ... now test yourself with key questions from the authors

- Go to the FastTest for this title
  FREE at **karger.com/fastfacts**
- Approximate time **10 minutes**
- For best retention of the key issues, try taking the FastTest before and after reading

Index